CARB CYCLING COOKBOOK FOR WOMEN

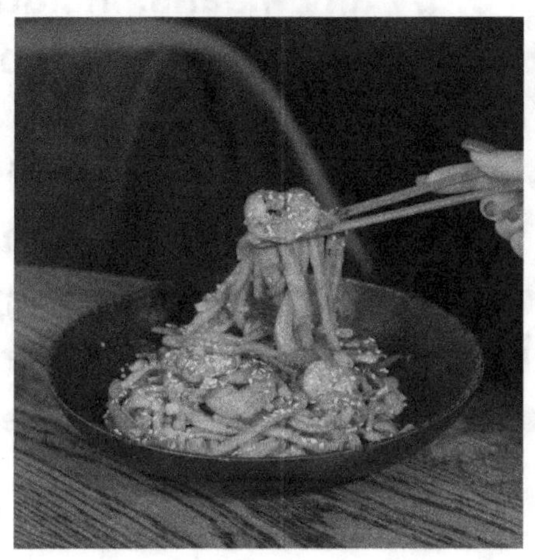

"Energize Your Lifestyle: A Carb Cycling Guide Tailored for Women's Health and Fitness with over 50 delicious recipes"

EMMA LYNCH

TABLE OF CONTENTS

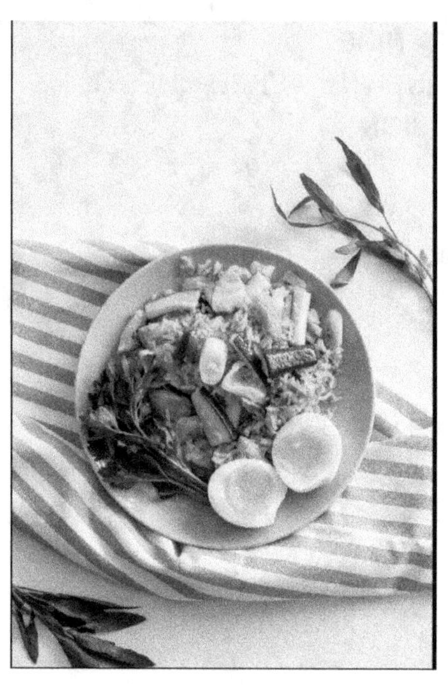

INTRODUCTION

Welcome to the "Carb Cycling Cookbook For Women" a comprehensive guide designed exclusively for women seeking a balanced and sustainable approach to nutrition and fitness. In the ever-evolving landscape of wellness, carb cycling emerges as a powerful tool, and this cookbook is your compass to navigate its benefits seamlessly.

In the pages ahead, we delve into the intricacies of carb cycling, exploring how this approach can optimize women's health, support fitness goals, and enhance overall well-being. Understanding the dynamic relationship between macronutrients becomes the cornerstone of our journey. We break down the roles of proteins, fats, and carbohydrates, providing insights into crafting personalized ratios that align with your unique physiology.

Getting started is made accessible through practical advice on assessing your fitness objectives and selecting the most suitable carb cycle. Whether your goal is weight management, muscle building, or simply sustaining energy levels, this cookbook offers tailored weekly meal plans with delicious recipes for high, low, and moderate carb days. Each section is crafted with the understanding that women's nutritional needs fluctuate throughout the month, embracing the natural ebb and flow of hormonal cycles.

Embark on a culinary adventure with our meticulously curated recipes, focusing on breakfast, lunch, dinner, and satisfying snacks and desserts. As you navigate the delectable array of options, discover nutritional tips, supplementation guidance, and insights into adjusting carb intake. "Carb Cycling Cookbook For Women" is more than a cookbook; it's a holistic companion on your path to revitalizing your lifestyle, empowering you to embrace the benefits of carb cycling with confidence and vitality.

CHAPTER ONE

UNDERSTANDING CARB CYCLING

Carb cycling is a nutritional strategy that involves alternating the intake of carbohydrates over a specified period. Tailored specifically for women, this approach recognizes and aligns with the unique hormonal fluctuations women experience throughout their menstrual cycle. By intelligently manipulating carbohydrate intake, carb cycling aims to optimize energy levels, support fitness goals, and enhance overall well-being.

1. Macronutrient Ratios:
   To comprehend carb cycling, it's essential to understand the role of macronutrients—proteins, fats, and carbohydrates. Proteins contribute to muscle repair and maintenance, fats play a crucial role in hormonal balance, and carbohydrates provide energy. Carb cycling involves adjusting the proportions of these macronutrients based on specific phases of your cycle or fitness objectives.

2. Hormonal Considerations:
   Hormone fluctuations occur naturally in women during their menstrual cycle. Carb cycling takes this into account by adapting carbohydrate intake to different phases. For example, during the follicular

phase, when estrogen is dominant, higher carbohydrate intake can support increased energy needs. In contrast, during the luteal phase, when progesterone rises, a moderate carbohydrate approach may be beneficial.

3. Fitness Goals and Carb Cycling:
Carb cycling can be tailored to various fitness goals, whether it's weight loss, muscle building, or maintaining overall health. Understanding how to align your carb cycle with your objectives ensures that you provide your body with the right fuel at the right times.

4. Metabolic Impact:
Carb cycling can influence metabolism by preventing adaptation to a consistently low-carbohydrate or high-carbohydrate diet. This strategic variation keeps the body responsive to different fuel sources, potentially enhancing fat utilization while preserving muscle mass.

5. Getting Started:
Assessing your fitness goals and understanding your menstrual cycle form the foundation of embarking on a carb cycling journey. This involves identifying the phases of your cycle, selecting the appropriate macronutrient ratios, and planning your carb cycle accordingly.

6. Personalization and Adaptation:

Carb cycling's versatility is one of its advantages. It's not a one-size-fits-all approach. As you progress, you may need to adjust your carb cycling plan based on how your body responds, ensuring that it continues to meet your evolving needs.

By comprehensively understanding carb cycling within the context of women's health, this cookbook empowers you to make informed choices, supporting your wellness journey with a flexible and effective nutritional strategy.

BENEFITS FOR WOMEN

Carb cycling offers a range of benefits specifically tailored to women's health and fitness:

1. Hormonal Balance:
Recognizing and adapting to the hormonal fluctuations in a woman's menstrual cycle, carb cycling can support hormonal balance. Aligning carbohydrate intake with different phases of the cycle may contribute to improved mood, energy levels, and overall well-being.

2. Energy Optimization:
Tailoring carbohydrate intake to match energy demands during specific phases of the menstrual cycle ensures that women have the necessary fuel for physical activities. This can enhance workout performance and daily energy levels.

3. Weight Management:

Carb cycling provides a flexible approach to calorie and carbohydrate manipulation, making it effective for weight management goals. By strategically adjusting carbohydrate intake, women can manage caloric intake based on their activity levels and metabolic needs.

4. Preserving Lean Muscle Mass:

The strategic variation in carbohydrate intake prevents the body from adapting to a consistent dietary pattern. This may help in preserving lean muscle mass, especially when combined with appropriate protein intake and strength training exercises.

5. Improved Insulin Sensitivity:

Cycling between higher and lower carbohydrate days can contribute to improved insulin sensitivity. This is particularly relevant for women, as insulin sensitivity plays a crucial role in managing blood sugar levels and supporting overall metabolic health.

6. Menstrual Cycle Support:

Carb cycling can be adapted to provide nutritional support during different phases of the menstrual cycle. Adjusting macronutrient ratios may help alleviate premenstrual symptoms and support energy levels during menstruation.

7. Flexibility and Sustainability:
   A versatile and sustainable approach to nutrition is provided by carb cycling. It allows for variations in food choices and can be adapted to accommodate different lifestyles, making it a practical long-term solution for women seeking nutritional balance.

8. Adaptable to Fitness Goals:
   Whether the goal is fat loss, muscle gain, or maintenance, carb cycling can be tailored to suit individual fitness objectives. This adaptability makes it a versatile strategy that can evolve with changing fitness goals over time.

Understanding and harnessing these benefits empower women to take charge of their nutritional choices, supporting a holistic approach to health and fitness through the principles of carb cycling.

HOW CARB CYCLING WORKS

Carb cycling operates on the principle of strategically varying carbohydrate intake over a specified period. This approach aims to optimize energy utilization, promote fat loss, preserve muscle mass, and align nutritional intake with specific goals or phases. Here's how carb cycling works:

1. Macronutrient Manipulation:

Carb cycling involves adjusting the proportions of macronutrients—proteins, fats, and carbohydrates—based on specific days or phases. High carb days typically involve increased carbohydrate intake, while low carb days restrict carbohydrate consumption. This variation aims to influence the body's metabolism and energy utilization.

2. Hormonal Adaptation:
Carb cycling takes into account hormonal fluctuations, especially in women's menstrual cycles. During different phases, such as the follicular and luteal phases, hormonal changes can affect energy needs and nutrient utilization. Adapting carbohydrate intake to these hormonal variations supports overall hormonal balance.

3. Glycogen Depletion and Refeeding:
Low carb days contribute to glycogen depletion, prompting the body to tap into stored fat for energy. This can be beneficial for those aiming for fat loss. On high carb days, glycogen stores are replenished, supporting energy levels and muscle recovery.

4. Insulin Sensitivity:
Alternating between low and high carb days may improve insulin sensitivity. Low carb days reduce the frequency of insulin spikes, while high carb days support the body's response to insulin.

Improved insulin sensitivity is associated with better blood sugar control and metabolic health.

5. Metabolic Flexibility:
Regularly changing carbohydrate intake prevents the body from adapting to a fixed dietary pattern. This promotes metabolic flexibility, enabling the body to efficiently switch between burning carbohydrates and fat for fuel.

6. Fitness Goals Alignment:
Carb cycling can be tailored to align with specific fitness goals. For instance, high carb days may support intense workout sessions, while low carb days can be scheduled during rest or lighter activity days. This customization ensures that nutritional intake complements the demands of different phases in a training program.

7. Individualization and Adaptation:
Carb cycling is not a one-size-fits-all approach. It requires observation and adaptation based on individual responses. Factors such as activity levels, metabolism, and personal preferences play a role in determining the most effective carb cycling strategy for an individual.

By strategically manipulating carbohydrate intake, carb cycling provides a dynamic and flexible approach to nutrition, allowing individuals to harness its benefits for improved energy, metabolism, and overall health.

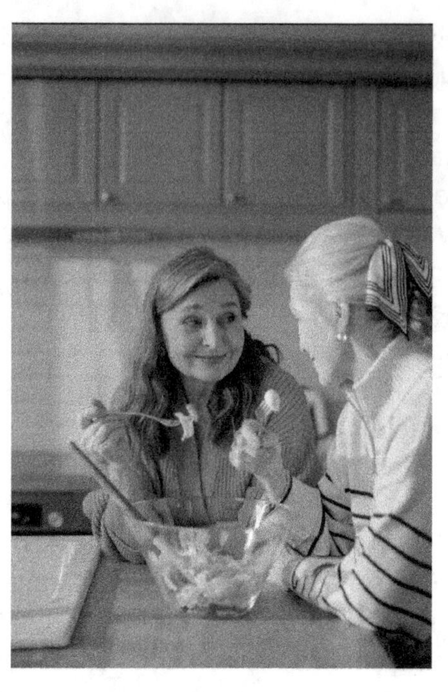

CHAPTER TWO

SETTING YOUR MACRONUTRIENT RATIOS

Setting macronutrient ratios is a crucial aspect of carb cycling, tailored to individual goals and preferences. Here's a guide to help you establish effective macronutrient ratios for carb cycling:

Determine Total Daily Caloric Intake

Determining your total daily caloric intake is a crucial step in creating a foundation for effective nutrition planning. Here's a simplified guide to help you calculate it:

1. **Calculate Basal Metabolic Rate (BMR):**
   - For women, you can use the Harris-Benedict equation:
   $$ BMR = 655 + (4.35 \times \text{weight in pounds}) + (4.7 \times \text{height in inches}) - (4.7 \times \text{age in years}) $$

2. **Factor in Physical Activity:**
   - To account for everyday activities and exercise, multiply your BMR by an activity factor.
   - Sedentary (little or no exercise): BMR $\times$ 1.2

- Lightly active (light exercise/sports 1-3 days/week): BMR $\times$ 1.375
- Moderately active (moderate exercise/sports 3-5 days/week): BMR $\times$ 1.55
- Very active (hard exercise/sports 6-7 days a week): BMR $\times$ 1.725
- Extremely active (very hard exercise/sports, physical job, or training twice a day): BMR $\times$ 1.9

3. **Set Goals:**
   - Adjust your total daily caloric intake based on your goals.
   - **For weight maintenance:** Maintain the calculated total.
   - **For weight loss:** Consume fewer calories than calculated, creating a calorie deficit.
   - **For weight gain:** Consume more calories than calculated, creating a calorie surplus.

Remember, these calculations provide estimates, and individual variations may exist. Regularly reassess your progress and adjust your caloric intake based on how your body responds to achieve your specific health and fitness goals.

Establish Protein Intake

Establishing an appropriate protein intake is crucial for muscle health, recovery, and overall well-being.

Here's a guideline to help determine your protein needs:

1. **Calculate Your Protein Needs:**
   - Aim for a protein intake within the range of 0.7 to 1 gram per pound of body weight.
   - If you're more sedentary or have specific health considerations, you might lean toward the lower end of the range. For those engaged in regular physical activity or strength training, consider the higher end.

2. **Consider Your Fitness Goals:**
   - Tailor your protein intake based on your fitness objectives. If your goal is muscle gain or intense training, opting for a higher protein intake within the recommended range may be beneficial.

3. **Distribute Protein Intake Across Meals:**
   - Spread your protein intake evenly across meals to optimize muscle protein synthesis throughout the day.
   - Aim for a balance between animal and plant-based protein sources to ensure a diverse array of essential amino acids.

4. **Adjust Based on Individual Response:**
   - Monitor how your body responds to your chosen protein intake. Factors such as energy levels, muscle recovery, and overall well-being can provide valuable insights.

- Be open to adjusting your protein intake based on individual needs and preferences.

5. **Consider Daily Activities:**
   - If you engage in intense workouts, consider increasing protein intake on those days to support muscle repair and recovery.
   - On rest days or lighter activity days, you might adjust protein intake accordingly.

6. **Include Protein in Every Meal:**
   - Incorporate protein-rich foods into every meal, such as lean meats, poultry, fish, eggs, dairy products, legumes, and plant-based protein sources.
   - Utilize protein supplements if needed, but prioritize whole food sources for optimal nutrient intake.

Remember that individual needs vary, and it may take some experimentation to find the protein intake that works best for you. Regularly assess your progress and adjust your protein intake as needed to align with your fitness goals and overall health.

Allocate Fats

Allocating fats in your diet is essential for various bodily functions, including hormone production, cell structure, and nutrient absorption. Here's a guide to help you determine and allocate fats in your daily intake:

1. **Determine Total Fat Intake:**
   - Allocate approximately 20-35% of your total daily caloric intake to fats. This range provides flexibility based on individual preferences, metabolic rate, and overall dietary goals.

2. **Choose Healthy Fat Sources:**
   - Prioritize sources of healthy fats, such as avocados, nuts, seeds, olive oil, fatty fish (like salmon and mackerel), and coconut oil. These fats contain essential fatty acids that support overall health.

3. **Consider Omega-3 Fatty Acids:**
   - Ensure an adequate intake of omega-3 fatty acids, which are beneficial for heart health and inflammation. Add walnuts, chia seeds, flaxseeds, and fatty fish to your diet.

4. **Balance Saturated and Unsaturated Fats:**
   - Aim for a balance between saturated and unsaturated fats. While saturated fats are not inherently harmful, it's beneficial to prioritize unsaturated fats for heart health.

5. **Distribute Fats Across Meals:**
   - Spread your fat intake across meals to support sustained energy and nutrient absorption throughout the day.

6. **Adjust Based on Dietary Preferences:**
   - Adjust the distribution of fats based on your dietary preferences and restrictions. For example, those following a plant-based diet may rely more on nuts, seeds, and plant oils.

7. **Monitor Portion Sizes:**
   - Because fats are high in calories, watch how much you eat. Balancing fat intake with other macronutrients helps maintain overall calorie goals.

8. **Be Flexible and Individualize:**
   - Recognize that individual preferences and metabolic responses vary. Be flexible in adjusting fat intake based on how your body responds and what aligns with your overall well-being.

Remember, fats are an essential component of a balanced diet, and choosing the right types and amounts contributes to optimal health. Regularly assess your dietary choices and make adjustments as needed to meet your specific goals and preferences.

Distribute Carbohydrates

Distributing carbohydrates strategically is a key aspect of carb cycling. Here's a guide to help you distribute carbohydrates in your diet based on different days or phases:

1. **High Carb Days:**
   - On days with higher activity levels or intense workouts, allocate around 45-65% of your total daily caloric intake to carbohydrates.
   - Choose complex carbohydrates like whole grains, sweet potatoes, legumes, and fruits for sustained energy.

2. **Low Carb Days:**
   - On rest days or days with lighter activity, reduce carbohydrate intake to approximately 10-30% of your total daily calories.
   - Focus on non-starchy vegetables, lean proteins, and healthy fats to support satiety.

3. **Moderate Carb Days:**
   - Reserve around 30-50% of your total daily caloric intake for carbohydrates on moderate activity days.
   - Include a balance of complex carbohydrates, proteins, and fats to meet your energy needs.

4. **Align with Fitness Goals:**
   - Customize carbohydrate distribution based on your fitness objectives. Adjusting carb intake can support muscle glycogen replenishment on high activity days and encourage fat utilization on low activity days.

5. **Consider Hormonal Phases:**

- For women, align carbohydrate intake with different phases of the menstrual cycle. During the follicular phase, when energy needs may be higher, lean towards higher carb intake. In the luteal phase, consider a moderate approach.

6. **Choose Nutrient-Dense Carbohydrates:**
- Prioritize nutrient-dense carbohydrate sources, such as whole grains, vegetables, fruits, and legumes, to ensure you're meeting your micronutrient needs.

7. **Spread Carbohydrates Across Meals:**
- Distribute carbohydrate intake evenly across meals to support stable blood sugar levels throughout the day.
- This approach helps avoid energy crashes and supports sustained energy for daily activities.

8. **Be Flexible and Listen to Your Body:**
- Be open to adjusting carbohydrate distribution based on individual responses, energy levels, and preferences.
- Pay attention to how your body feels and performs, and make adjustments accordingly.

Remember, carb cycling allows for flexibility and adaptability. Experiment with different ratios and observe how your body responds to find the distribution that best aligns with your goals and well-being. Regularly reassess and make adjustments as needed.

Align with Fitness Goals

Aligning carbohydrate intake with your fitness goals is a crucial aspect of optimizing performance, energy levels, and overall well-being. Here's how you can tailor your carbohydrate consumption based on different fitness objectives:

1. **Muscle Building and Intense Workouts:**
   - On days with intense resistance training or high-intensity workouts, consider higher carbohydrate intake (45-65% of total calories).
   - Prioritize complex carbohydrates such as whole grains, oats, and sweet potatoes to replenish glycogen stores and support muscle recovery.

2. **Weight Loss and Low-Intensity Days:**
   - On days with lower activity levels or during weight loss phases, opt for a lower carbohydrate intake (10-30% of total calories).
   - Focus on non-starchy vegetables, lean proteins, and healthy fats to promote fat utilization for energy.

3. **Endurance Training:**
   - For endurance activities like long-distance running or cycling, moderate to high carbohydrate intake (30-50% of total calories) can help sustain energy levels.

- Include a mix of complex carbohydrates, proteins, and healthy fats to support endurance and prevent energy depletion.

4. **Adapt to Training Phases:**
   - Adjust carbohydrate intake based on different training phases, such as bulking, cutting, or maintenance.
   - During muscle-building phases, prioritize higher carbohydrate days to support energy needs and recovery.

5. **Post-Workout Nutrition:**
   - Schedule higher carbohydrate intake around your workout, especially during the post-workout period.
   - Including carbohydrates in this window helps replenish glycogen stores and supports efficient recovery.

6. **Hormonal Considerations:**
   - For women, align carbohydrate intake with hormonal phases. During the follicular phase (first half of the menstrual cycle), higher carbohydrate intake may align with increased energy needs.

7. **Monitor and Adjust:**
   - Regularly assess your energy levels, workout performance, and overall progress.
   - Be open to adjusting carbohydrate intake based on individual responses and changes in fitness goals.

8. **Maintain Balance:**
   - Strive for a balanced approach that includes all macronutrients. Carbohydrates, proteins, and fats each play a vital role in supporting overall fitness and health.

Remember that individual responses vary, and the optimal carbohydrate intake for one person may differ from another. Experiment with different approaches, observe how your body reacts, and make adjustments to find the carbohydrate distribution that aligns with your specific fitness objectives and preferences.

Consider Hormonal Phases

Considering hormonal phases, especially for women, is a crucial aspect of tailoring nutrition to support overall well-being and fitness goals. Here's how you can align carbohydrate intake with different hormonal phases:

1. **Follicular Phase (Days 1-14):**
   - During the follicular phase, which begins with the start of menstruation, estrogen levels rise, and energy expenditure tends to increase.
   - Consider incorporating higher carbohydrate intake (45-65% of total calories) during this phase to support increased energy needs.

2. **Ovulatory Phase (Days 15-17):**
   - Estrogen continues to rise, reaching its peak during ovulation. This phase may also see an increase in energy expenditure.
   - Maintain a moderate to higher carbohydrate intake, similar to the follicular phase, to support sustained energy levels.

3. **Luteal Phase (Days 18-28):**
   - Progesterone rises during the luteal phase, leading to potential changes in mood, increased cravings, and higher basal body temperature.
   - Consider a moderate carbohydrate intake (30-50% of total calories) during this phase. Focus on complex carbohydrates to help manage cravings and support energy levels.

4. **Menstruation (Varies):**
   - Individual responses to menstruation vary. Some may experience increased cravings and energy needs during this time.
   - Adjust carbohydrate intake based on individual comfort and energy requirements. For some, maintaining a balanced approach may work, while others may benefit from slight adjustments.

5. **Fluid Intake and Hydration:**
   - Stay well-hydrated throughout the menstrual cycle, as fluid needs may vary. Adequate hydration supports overall health and can help alleviate bloating and discomfort.

6. **Individual Observation:**
   - Pay attention to your body's signals, energy levels, and cravings throughout the menstrual cycle.
   - Adjust carbohydrate intake based on how your body responds, aiming for a balance between meeting energy needs and supporting hormonal fluctuations.

7. **Nutrient-Dense Choices:**
   - Emphasize nutrient-dense carbohydrates from whole grains, fruits, and vegetables throughout the menstrual cycle to ensure a broad spectrum of essential nutrients.

8. **Consult with Healthcare Professionals:**
   - If you have specific concerns or experience irregularities in your menstrual cycle, it's advisable to consult with healthcare professionals or nutrition experts for personalized guidance.

Adapting carbohydrate intake to hormonal phases is a dynamic approach that recognizes the unique needs and fluctuations in energy expenditure throughout the menstrual cycle. By aligning nutrition with hormonal changes, you can optimize energy levels, manage cravings, and support overall health and fitness goals.

Monitor and Adjust:

Monitoring and adjusting your nutrition plan is a critical component of achieving your health and fitness goals. Here's a guide on how to effectively monitor and make necessary adjustments:

1. **Regular Self-Assessment:**
   - Consistently assess how your body feels, your energy levels, and your overall well-being. Be mindful of any changes in mood, performance, or cravings.

2. **Performance Tracking:**
   - Keep a log of your workout performance, noting any changes in strength, endurance, or recovery. This can provide insights into how well your nutrition plan is supporting your fitness goals.

3. **Body Composition Changes:**
   - Track changes in body composition, such as weight, body fat percentage, and muscle mass. This can help you understand how your nutrition plan is influencing your physical progress.

4. **Energy Levels:**
   - Monitor your energy levels throughout the day. If you consistently feel fatigued or experience energy crashes, it may be an indication that adjustments to your macronutrient distribution are needed.

5. **Cravings and Hunger:**

- Pay attention to cravings and hunger signals. If you find yourself consistently craving certain foods or feeling excessively hungry, it could be a sign that your nutritional intake needs modification.

6. **Digestive Health:**
- Assess your digestive health. Any discomfort, bloating, or irregularities may suggest that certain foods or proportions in your diet need adjustment.

7. **Adapt to Changing Goals:**
- If your fitness goals change over time, such as transitioning from weight loss to muscle building, be prepared to adjust your macronutrient ratios accordingly.

8. **Be Flexible:**
- Recognize that your body's needs may change due to factors such as stress, sleep, and activity levels. Be flexible in adjusting your nutrition plan based on these dynamic variables.

9. **Consultation with Professionals:**
- If you're uncertain about the adjustments to make or encounter challenges, consider consulting with nutritionists, dietitians, or fitness professionals for personalized guidance.

10. **Trial and Error:**
- Understand that finding the optimal nutrition plan is often a process of trial and error. Experiment with different approaches, observe the outcomes,

and refine your plan based on what works best for you.

Remember, your nutrition plan is a dynamic aspect of your overall wellness journey. Regularly monitoring and adjusting it allows you to fine-tune your approach, ensuring that it continues to align with your evolving goals and supports your well-being effectively.

Stay Hydrated and Nutrient-Dense

Staying hydrated and consuming nutrient-dense foods are fundamental principles for supporting overall health and well-being. Here's a guide on how to prioritize hydration and nutrient density in your diet:

1. Hydration Guidelines:
  - Aim to drink at least 8 glasses (64 ounces) of water per day, but individual needs may vary based on factors like activity level, climate, and personal health.
  - Carry a reusable water bottle to make it easy to track and meet your daily water intake goals.

2. Nutrient-Dense Food Choices:
  - Prioritize whole, minimally processed foods that are rich in essential nutrients. These consist of whole grains, fruits, vegetables, lean meats, and healthy fats.

- Choose a variety of colorful fruits and vegetables to ensure a diverse range of vitamins, minerals, and antioxidants.

3. Balanced Macronutrients:
   - Include a balance of macronutrients (carbohydrates, proteins, and fats) in each meal to provide sustained energy and support various bodily functions.
   - Opt for complex carbohydrates, lean proteins, and healthy fats to enhance nutrient density.

4. Eat a Rainbow:
   - Consume a variety of fruits and vegetables of different colors to ensure a broad spectrum of nutrients. Each color represents unique phytonutrients with specific health benefits.

5. Limit Added Sugars and Processed Foods:
   - Minimize the intake of foods and beverages high in added sugars and heavily processed items.
   - Check food labels for hidden sugars and opt for whole, natural alternatives.

6. Include Lean Proteins:
   - Incorporate lean protein sources such as poultry, fish, beans, legumes, tofu, and low-fat dairy into your meals. Protein is necessary for both general satiety and the health of muscles.

7. Healthy Fats:

- Select foods like avocados, almonds, seeds, and olive oil that are high in healthful fats. These fats contribute to heart health and support nutrient absorption.

8. Hydrating Foods:
   - Consume hydrating foods like watermelon, cucumber, celery, and citrus fruits. These foods contribute to overall hydration and provide additional nutrients.

9. Listen to Your Body:
   - Pay attention to your body's signals for thirst and hunger. Often, thirst is mistaken for hunger, so staying adequately hydrated can help manage unnecessary snacking.

10. Moderation and Balance:
   - Embrace a balanced and moderate approach to your diet. Avoid extreme restrictions, and focus on creating a sustainable and enjoyable eating plan.

11. Consult with Professionals:
   - See a qualified dietitian or other healthcare provider for individualized guidance if you have any specific dietary questions or medical issues.

Prioritizing hydration and nutrient density supports your body's functions, energy levels, and overall health. By making mindful choices and incorporating a variety of nutrient-rich foods, you can create a foundation for long-term well-being.

Remember, individual responses vary, so it's essential to observe how your body reacts and make adjustments accordingly. Consistency and flexibility in adjusting macronutrient ratios will help you tailor carb cycling to your specific needs and maximize its benefits.

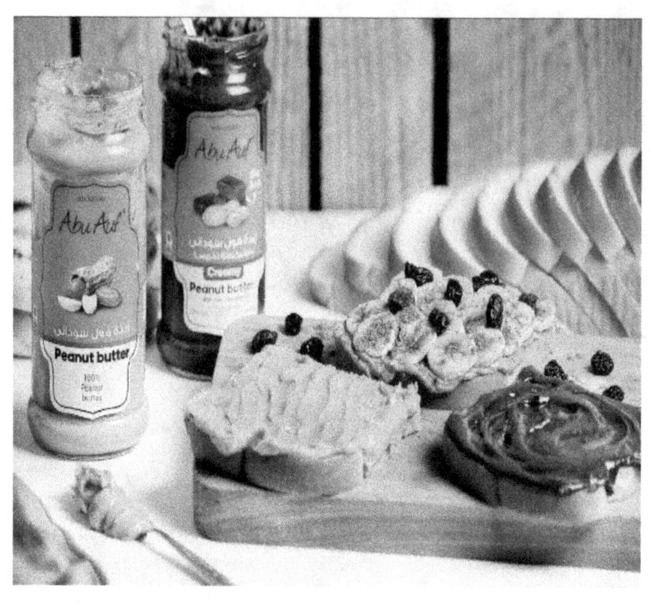
AbuAli
Peanut butter
زبدة فول سوداني
Peanut butter
100%
Peanut
butter
AbuAli
Peanut butter

CHAPTER THREE

WEEKLY MEAL PLANS

Creating a weekly meal plan is a great way to stay organized, save time, and ensure you're meeting your nutritional goals. Here's a sample weekly meal plan incorporating carb cycling principles. Adjust portions and specific foods based on your preferences, dietary restrictions, and caloric needs.

Day 1: High Carb Day (Workout Day)

Breakfast:
- Oatmeal with almond butter and banana
- Greek yogurt with honey and almonds

Lunch:
- Sweet potatoe and black bean bowl
- Steamed broccoli on the side

Snack:
- Banana and almond toast

Dinner:
- chicken and broccoli Alfredo
- Turkey and vegetable skillet
- Mixed green salad with a variety of veggies

Day 2: Low Carb Day (Rest or Light Activity Day)

Breakfast:
- Spinach and feta omelette
- Avocado slices

Lunch:
- Grilled chicken salad
- Cauliflower fried rice with vegetables and tofu

Snack:
- Cucumber and cream cheese bites

Dinner:
- Baked lemon herb chicken
- Grilled Salmon with avocado salsa
- Eggplant lasagna

Day 3: Moderate Carb Day (Moderate Activity Day)

Breakfast:
- Whole grain toast with smashed avocado
- Mixed berries

Lunch:
- chickpea and avocado wrap
- Side of sliced cucumber

Snack:
- Apple slices with a small handful of almonds

Dinner:
- Turkey and vegetable quinoa bowl
- Salmon and asparagus bake
- Shrimp and broccoli Stir-Fry

Repeat the pattern, alternating between high, low, and moderate carb days based on your activity levels and fitness goals. Customize the plan by incorporating a variety of protein sources, healthy fats, and fiber-rich carbohydrates. Adjust portion sizes to match your caloric needs and monitor your progress to make any necessary tweaks to the meal plan. Always consult with a healthcare or nutrition professional if you have specific dietary concerns or health conditions.

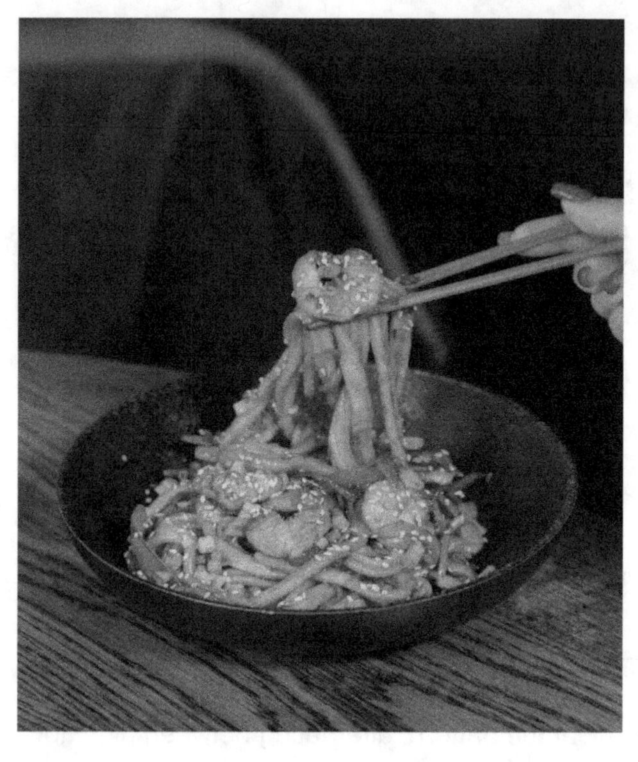

CHAPTER FOUR

RECIPES FOR HIGH CARB DAYS

BREAKFAST

Certainly! Here are five breakfast recipes suitable for high carb days:

Berry Banana Smoothie Bowl

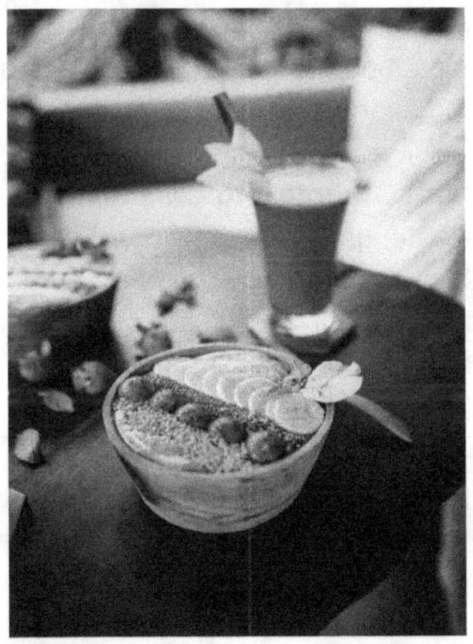

Ingredients:
- 1 frozen banana
- One cup of mixed berries, including raspberries, blueberries, and strawberries

- 1/2 cup Greek yogurt
- 1/4 cup granola
- 1 tablespoon chia seeds
- Honey (optional, for drizzling)

Instructions:
1. **Prepare the Smoothie Base:**
   - In a blender, combine the frozen banana, mixed berries, and Greek yogurt.
   - Blend until smooth and creamy. Add a splash of water or milk if needed to reach your desired consistency.

2. **Pour into a Bowl:**
   - Pour the smoothie into a bowl, ensuring a smooth and even surface.

3. **Top with Granola and Chia Seeds:**
   - Sprinkle the granola evenly over the smoothie surface to create a crunchy texture.
   - Add a tablespoon of chia seeds for added nutrition and texture.

4. **Decorate with Fresh Berries:**
   - Arrange additional fresh berries (strawberries, blueberries, raspberries) on top of the granola for a burst of color and flavor.

5. **Drizzle with Honey (Optional):**
   - If you have a sweet tooth, drizzle honey over the entire bowl for a touch of natural sweetness.

6. **Serve and Enjoy:**
   - Grab a spoon and enjoy your delicious and nutrient-packed Berry Banana Smoothie Bowl!

Nutritional Value (Approx. per Serving):

Calories: 300
Protein: 12g
Fat: 8g
Carbohydrates: 45g

Feel free to customize this recipe by adding your favorite toppings such as sliced almonds, coconut flakes, or extra fruit. This smoothie bowl is not only visually appealing but also a great way to kickstart your high carb day with a mix of carbohydrates, healthy fats, and protein.

Whole Grain Pancakes with Fruit

Ingredients:
- 1 cup whole grain pancake mix
- 1 cup milk (or plant-based alternative)
- 1 egg
- Mixed fresh fruit (berries, sliced bananas)
- Maple syrup

Instructions:

1. **Prepare the Pancake Batter:**

- In a bowl, mix the whole grain pancake mix, milk, and egg until well combined. If necessary, adjust the consistency by adding extra milk.

2. **Heat the Griddle or Pan:**
- Preheat a griddle or non-stick pan over medium heat. Apply a small bit of oil or cooking spray to the surface to lightly coat it.

3. **Cook the Pancakes:**
- Pour 1/4 cup of pancake batter onto the griddle for each pancake.
- cook until surface bubbles appear, then turn and continue cooking until the other side becomes golden brown.

4. **Repeat:**
- Repeat the process until you have a stack of delicious whole grain pancakes.

5. **Serve with Fresh Fruit:**
- Arrange mixed fresh fruit, such as berries and sliced bananas, on top of the pancake stack.

6. **Drizzle with Maple Syrup:**
- Finish by drizzling maple syrup over the pancakes and fruit.

7. **Optional Extras:**
- Sprinkle with chopped nuts or a dusting of cinnamon for added flavor and texture.

8. **Enjoy:**
   - Grab a fork and enjoy a wholesome and tasty
breakfast with the goodness of whole grains and
fresh fruit.

Nutritional Value (Approx. per Serving):

Calories: 300
Protein: 8g
Fat: 5g
Carbohydrates: 60g

Feel free to get creative with your fruit toppings,
and consider adding a dollop of Greek yogurt for an
extra protein boost. This breakfast is a delightful
way to start your high carb day with a balance of
complex carbohydrates, natural sugars, and
essential nutrients.

Oatmeal with Almond Butter and Banana

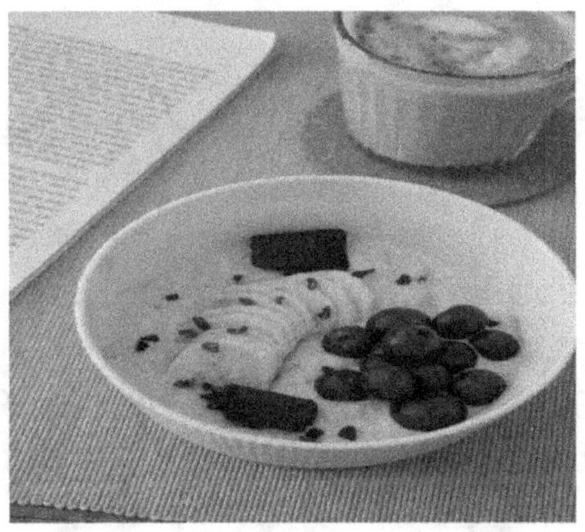

Ingredients:
- 1/2 cup rolled oats
- 1 cup milk (or water)
- 1 banana, sliced
- 1 tablespoon almond butter
- Chopped nuts (optional)

Instructions:

1. **Cook the Oats:**
   - Place the rolled oats and milk (or water) in a saucepan. Cook over medium heat, stirring occasionally, until the oats are creamy and have absorbed the liquid.

2. **Slice the Banana:**
   - While the oats are cooking, slice the banana into rounds.

3. **Assemble the Oatmeal:**
   - Once the oats are cooked, transfer them to a bowl.

4. **Add Banana Slices:**
   - Arrange the banana slices on top of the oatmeal.

5. **Drizzle with Almond Butter:**
   - Spoon almond butter over the banana slices. The warmth of the oats will help the almond butter melt slightly.

6. **Optional: Add Chopped Nuts:**
   - If desired, sprinkle with chopped nuts (such as almonds or walnuts) for added crunch and nutrition.

7. **Mix and Enjoy:**
   - To combine the flavors, gently mix the ingredients together.

8. **Serve Warm:**
   - Enjoy your comforting bowl of Oatmeal with Almond Butter and Banana while it's warm.

Nutritional Value (Approx. per Serving):

Calories: 400
Protein: 12g
Fat: 18g
Carbohydrates: 55g

This breakfast is not only delicious but also provides a mix of complex carbohydrates, healthy fats, and natural sweetness from the banana. It's a satisfying way to fuel your high carb day with nutrient-dense ingredients.

Whole Wheat Toast with Avocado and Poached Eggs

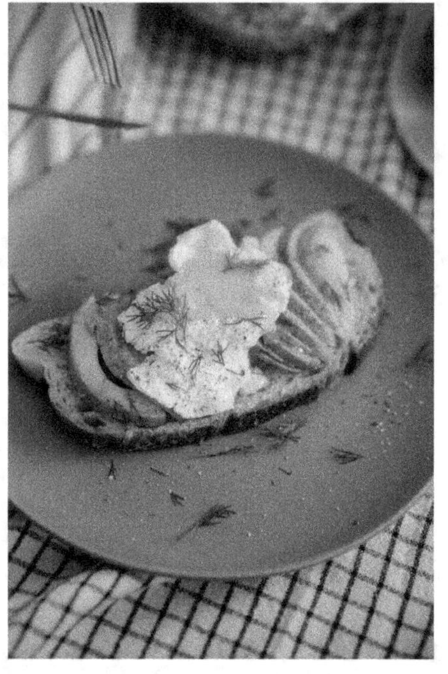

Ingredients:

- 2 slices whole wheat bread, toasted
- 1 ripe avocado, mashed
- 2 poached eggs
- Salt and pepper to taste
- Red pepper flakes (optional)

Instructions:

1. **Toast the Bread:**

- Toast two slices of whole wheat bread until golden brown.

2. **Mash the Avocado:**
   - Mash the ripe avocado in a bowl while the bread is toasting. To taste, add salt and pepper.

3. **Poach the Eggs:**
   - Poach two eggs using your preferred method. For a classic poached egg, bring water to a simmer, add a splash of vinegar, and gently slide each egg into the simmering water. Cook until the yolks are still runny but the whites are set.

4. **Assemble the Toast:**
   - Spread the mashed avocado evenly on each slice of toasted bread.

5. **Top with Poached Eggs:**
   - Carefully place a poached egg on top of each slice of avocado-covered toast.

6. **Season to Taste:**
   - Sprinkle it with additional salt and pepper to taste. If you like a bit of heat, add red pepper flakes for some spice.

7. **Optional Garnish:**
   - Garnish with fresh herbs like chopped chives or cilantro for added flavor and freshness.

8. **Serve Immediately:**

- Serve your Whole Wheat Toast with Avocado
and Poached Eggs immediately, while the eggs are
warm and the toast is crispy.

Nutritional Value (Approx. per Serving):

Calories: 300
Protein: 15g
Fat: 15g
Carbohydrates: 25g

This breakfast combines the creaminess of
avocado with the richness of poached eggs on
wholesome whole wheat toast. It's a balanced and
nutritious way to start your high carb day with a mix
of healthy fats, protein, and complex
carbohydrates.

Greek Yogurt With Honey and Almonds

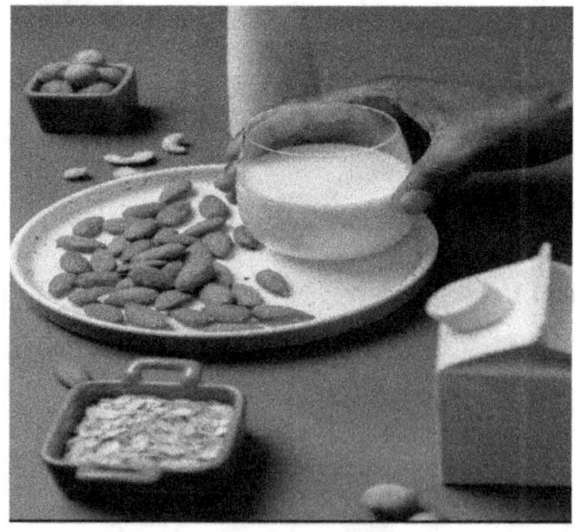

Ingredients:
- 1 cup Greek yogurt
- 1 tablespoon honey
- 2 tablespoons almonds, sliced or chopped

Instructions:

1. **Prepare the Greek Yogurt:**
   - Scoop one cup of Greek yogurt into a serving bowl.

2. **Drizzle with Honey:**
   - Drizzle honey evenly over the Greek yogurt. Depending on your preferred level of sweetness, adjust the amount of honey.

3. **Sprinkle with Almonds:**
   - Sprinkle sliced or chopped almonds on top of the Greek yogurt and honey.

4. **Optional: Add Extra Toppings:**
   - Enhance the flavor and texture by adding extras like a sprinkle of cinnamon, a handful of fresh berries, or a few granola clusters.

5. **Mix Gently (Optional):**
   - If you prefer, gently mix the honey, almonds, and any additional toppings into the Greek yogurt.

6. **Serve Immediately:**

  - Enjoy your delicious Greek Yogurt with Honey and Almonds immediately for a creamy, sweet, and crunchy breakfast or snack.

Nutritional Value (Approx. per Serving):

Calories: 250
Protein: 15g
Fat: 12g
Carbohydrates: 20g

This simple yet satisfying combination provides a balance of protein, healthy fats, and natural sweetness. It's a quick and nutritious option for your high carb day, offering a blend of textures and flavors to kickstart your day or provide a tasty energy boost.

You are welcome to alter these recipes to suit your dietary requirements and preferences. Enjoy your high carb breakfasts!

LUNCH

Certainly! Here are five lunch recipes suitable for high carb days, providing a good balance of carbohydrates, proteins, and healthy fats:

Quinoa and Vegetable Stir-Fry

Ingredients:
- 1 cup cooked quinoa
- mixed veggies, including broccoli, snap peas, and bell peppers
- Tofu or chicken, diced
- Soy sauce
- Sesame oil
- Garlic and ginger, minced
- Sesame seeds for garnish

Instructions:

1. **Prepare Quinoa:**
   - Cook quinoa according to package instructions. Set aside.

2. **Stir-Fry Tofu or Chicken:**
   - In a large pan or wok, stir-fry diced tofu or chicken in sesame oil over medium-high heat until cooked through and slightly browned.

3. **Add Garlic and Ginger:**
   - Add minced garlic and ginger to the pan. Stir-fry until aromatic, about one to two minutes.

4. **Cook Mixed Vegetables:**
   - Add mixed vegetables (bell peppers, broccoli, snap peas, or any of your choice) to the pan. Stir-fry until the vegetables are crisp-tender.

5. **Combine Quinoa:**
   - Add the cooked quinoa to the pan, mixing it with the tofu or chicken and vegetables.

6. **Season with Soy Sauce:**
   - Drizzle soy sauce over the quinoa and vegetable mixture. Toss everything together until well coated.

7. **Garnish and Serve:**
   - Sprinkle sesame seeds over the stir-fry for added texture and flavor.
   - Serve the Quinoa and Vegetable Stir-Fry hot, and enjoy a delicious and nutritious high carb meal.

Nutritional Value (Approx. per Serving):

Calories: 400
Protein: 20g
Fat: 10g
Carbohydrates: 60g

Feel free to customize this recipe by adding your favorite vegetables or adjusting the level of soy sauce to your taste preference. It's a versatile and quick stir-fry that provides a good balance of carbohydrates, protein, and vegetables.

Chickpea and Sweet Potato Curry

Ingredients:
- 1 can chickpeas, drained and rinsed
- 1 large sweet potato, diced
- Coconut milk
- Curry powder, cumin, and turmeric
- Spinach or kale
- Basmati rice

Instructions:

1. **Sauté Sweet Potatoes:**
   - In a pot, sauté diced sweet potatoes with curry powder, cumin, and turmeric in a bit of oil until they begin to soften.

2. **Add Coconut Milk:**
   - Pour in coconut milk, enough to cover the sweet potatoes. Bring to a simmer.

3. **Introduce Chickpeas:**
   - Stir in drained and rinsed chickpeas. Let the mixture simmer until sweet potatoes are tender and chickpeas are heated through.

4. **Season to Taste:**
   - Adjust the seasoning with additional curry powder, cumin, or turmeric as needed. Add salt and pepper to taste.

5. **Add Greens:**
   - Just before serving, stir in a handful of spinach or kale until wilted.

6. **Prepare Basmati Rice:**
   - While the curry is simmering, cook basmati rice according to package instructions.

7. **Serve:**
   - Spoon the chickpea and sweet potato curry over a bed of basmati rice.

8. **Optional Garnish:**
   - For added taste, add some fresh cilantro and a squeeze of lime juice.

Nutritional Value (Approx. per Serving):

Calories: 450
Protein: 15g
Fat: 15g
Carbohydrates: 65g

This Chickpea and Sweet Potato Curry is a hearty and flavorful high carb dish that combines the sweetness of sweet potatoes with the earthy taste of chickpeas and the rich creaminess of coconut milk. It's perfect for satisfying your cravings on high carb days.

Grilled Chicken and Quinoa Salad

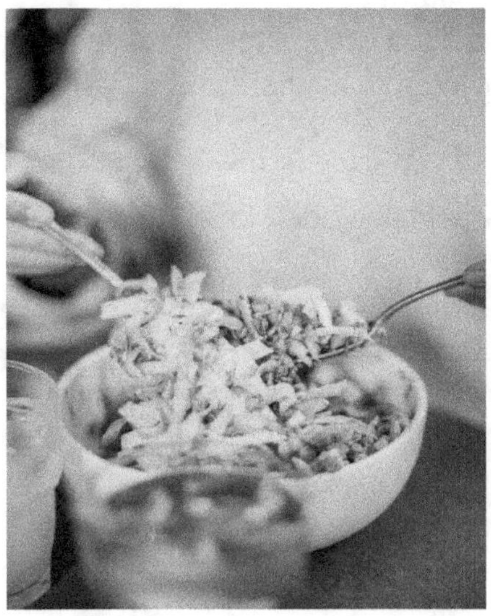

Ingredients:

- Grilled chicken breast, sliced
- 1 cup cooked quinoa
- Mixed greens
- Cherry tomatoes, halved
- Cucumber, sliced
- Feta cheese
- Balsamic vinaigrette

Instructions:

1. **Prepare Grilled Chicken:**
   - Grill chicken breast until fully cooked. Allow it to rest before slicing into strips.

2. **Cook Quinoa:**
   - Cook quinoa according to package instructions.
Let it cool to room temperature.

3. **Assemble the Salad:**
   - In a large salad bowl, layer mixed greens as the
base.

4. **Add Quinoa:**
   - Spoon cooked quinoa over the mixed greens.

5. **Top with Vegetables:**
   - Arrange halved cherry tomatoes and sliced
cucumber over the quinoa.

6. **Add Grilled Chicken:**
   - Arrange the grilled chicken slices over the salad.

7. **Sprinkle with Feta Cheese:**
   - Sprinkle crumbled feta cheese over the salad for
a creamy touch.

8. **Drizzle with Balsamic Vinaigrette:**
   - Drizzle balsamic vinaigrette dressing over the
salad. You can choose how much or how little to
use.

9. **Toss Gently:**
   - To equally distribute the ingredients and coat
them with the dressing, gently toss the salad.

10. **Serve Immediately:**

   - Serve the Grilled Chicken and Quinoa Salad immediately, providing a satisfying and balanced high carb meal.

Nutritional Value (Approx. per Serving):

Calories: 480
Protein: 35g
Fat: 20g
Carbohydrates: 40g

Feel free to customize this salad by adding other vegetables, nuts, or your favorite dressing. This dish offers a combination of lean protein from the grilled chicken, the nutritional goodness of quinoa, and the freshness of colorful vegetables for a delightful and nutritious high carb lunch.

Lentil and Vegetable Wrap

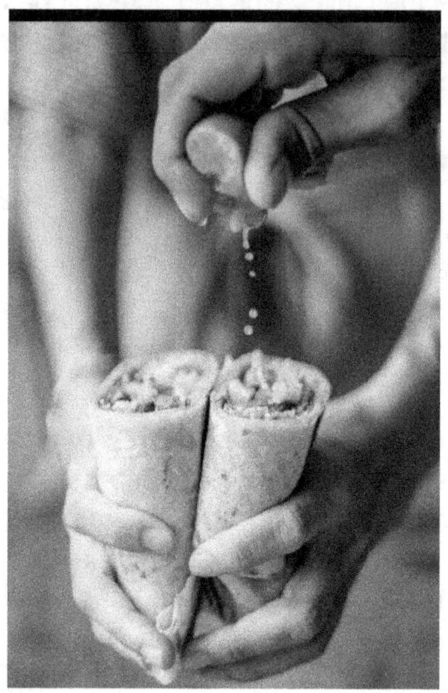

Ingredients:

- Whole grain wraps
- Cooked lentils
- Hummus
- Spinach or lettuce
- Cherry tomatoes, sliced
- Red onion, thinly sliced
- Feta cheese (optional)

Instructions:

1. **Prepare Lentils:**
   - Cook lentils according to package instructions until they are tender but still hold their shape. Allow them to cool.

2. **Warm the Wraps:**
   - Warm the whole grain wraps in a dry skillet or microwave for a few seconds to make them pliable.

3. **Spread Hummus:**
   - Spread a generous layer of hummus onto each wrap, leaving a border around the edges.

4. **Layer with Lentils:**
   - Spoon cooked lentils onto the hummus-covered area of the wraps.

5. **Add Vegetables:**
   - Layer with fresh spinach or lettuce, sliced cherry tomatoes, and thinly sliced red onion.

6. **Optional Feta Cheese:**
   - If desired, crumble feta cheese on top for an extra burst of flavor.

7. **Fold and Roll:**
   - Fold the sides of the wraps inward, then roll them tightly from the bottom, creating a secure wrap.

8. **Slice in Half (Optional):**

  - If you prefer, slice the wraps in half diagonally for easier handling.

9. **Serve:**
  - Serve the Lentil and Vegetable Wraps immediately, or pack them for a delicious and portable high carb lunch.

Nutritional Value (Approx. per Serving):

Calories: 380
Protein: 18g
Fat: 12g
Carbohydrates: 55g

Feel free to experiment with additional ingredients like cucumbers, bell peppers, or a drizzle of balsamic glaze. This versatile and plant-based wrap is a fantastic way to incorporate lentils and a variety of colorful vegetables into your high carb day.

Sweet Potato and Black Bean Bowl

Ingredients:

- Roasted sweet potatoes
- Black beans, cooked
- Brown rice or quinoa
- Avocado, sliced

- Salsa
- Lime wedges

Instructions:

1. **Roast Sweet Potatoes:**
   - Preheat the oven to 400°F (200°C). Toss peeled and diced sweet potatoes in olive oil, salt, and pepper. Roast until tender and slightly caramelized.

2. **Cook Black Beans:**
   - If using canned black beans, rinse and drain them. If using dried beans, cook them according to package instructions.

3. **Prepare Brown Rice or Quinoa:**
   - Cook brown rice or quinoa according to package instructions.

4. **Assemble the Bowl:**
   - In individual bowls, layer cooked brown rice or quinoa as the base.

5. **Add Sweet Potatoes and Black Beans:**
   - Top with roasted sweet potatoes and cooked black beans.

6. **Slice Avocado:**
   - Slice avocado and arrange it on top of the bowl.

7. **Drizzle with Salsa:**

   - Drizzle your favorite salsa over the bowl for a burst of flavor.

8. **Squeeze Lime Wedges:**
   - Finish by squeezing lime wedges over the entire bowl for a refreshing citrus touch.

9. **Optional Garnish:**
   - If desired, garnish with green onions or cilantro.

10. **Serve:**
   - Serve the Sweet Potato and Black Bean Bowl immediately, offering a nutritious and delicious high carb meal.

Nutritional Value (Approx. per Serving):

Calories: 420
Protein: 15g
Fat: 15g
Carbohydrates: 60g

Feel free to customize this bowl by adding other vegetables, a dollop of Greek yogurt, or a sprinkle of cheese. This colorful and nutrient-rich dish provides a mix of complex carbohydrates, protein, and healthy fats for a satisfying high carb lunch.

They provide a mix of whole grains, lean proteins, and plenty of colorful vegetables for a satisfying high carb lunch.

DINNER

Certainly! Here are five dinner recipes for high carb days, each providing a balance of macronutrients:

Chicken and Broccoli Alfredo

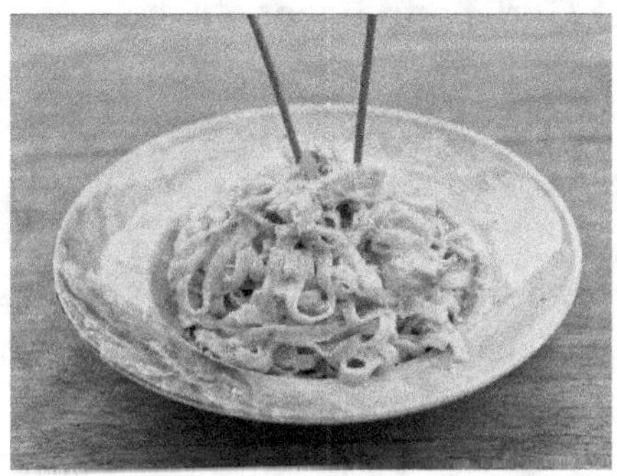

Ingredients:
- Grilled chicken breast, sliced
- 2 cups broccoli florets
- Whole wheat fettuccine pasta
- Alfredo sauce
- Parmesan cheese
- Garlic, minced
- Olive oil
- Salt and pepper to taste

Instructions:

1. **Cook Whole Wheat Fettuccine:**

- Cook the whole wheat fettuccine pasta according to the package instructions. Drain and set aside.

2. **Grill Chicken:**
   - Grill chicken breast until fully cooked. Before slicing into strips, let it rest for a few minutes.

3. **Sauté Garlic and Broccoli:**
   - Minced garlic should be cooked in olive oil until aromatic in a big pan. Cook the broccoli florets until they become crisp-tender.

4. **Combine Chicken, Broccoli, and Pasta:**
   - Add the sliced grilled chicken to the pan with the broccoli and garlic. Mix well.

5. **Pour Alfredo Sauce:**
   - Pour Alfredo sauce over the chicken, broccoli, and pasta mixture. Stir until the ingredients are coated evenly.

6. **Season to Taste:**
   - Add pepper and salt to taste. Be mindful of the salt content in the Alfredo sauce.

7. **Sprinkle with Parmesan:**
   - Sprinkle grated Parmesan cheese over the chicken and broccoli Alfredo. Stir to incorporate.

8. **Serve:**

- Serve the Chicken and Broccoli Alfredo over whole wheat fettuccine, ensuring a balanced combination of protein, vegetables, and complex carbohydrates.

9. **Garnish (Optional):**
- Optionally, garnish with additional Parmesan cheese and freshly chopped parsley for added flavor.

Nutritional Value (Approx. per Serving):

Calories: 550
Protein: 30g
Fat: 25g
Carbohydrates: 45g

This wholesome and tasty dish provides a nutritious blend of grilled chicken, fiber-rich whole wheat pasta, and nutrient-packed broccoli, all coated in a creamy Alfredo sauce. Enjoy your high carb meal!

Beef and Vegetable Stir-Fry

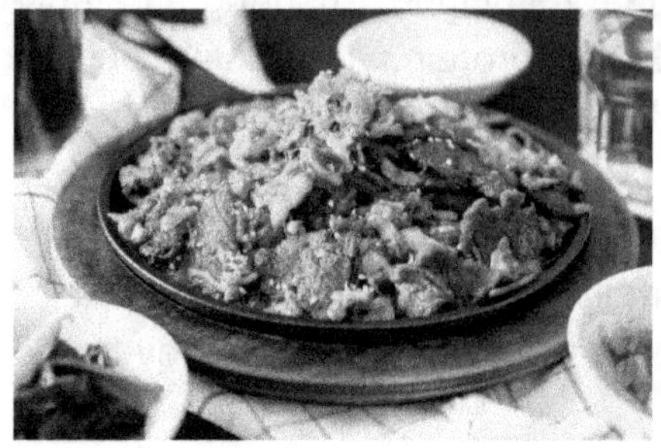

Ingredients:
- Thinly sliced beef strips
- Variety of vegetables (carrots, snap peas, and bell peppers)
- Brown rice
- Soy sauce
- Ginger, minced
- Garlic, minced
- Sesame oil
- Olive oil
- Green onions for garnish

Instructions:

1. **Cook Brown Rice:**
   - Brown rice should be cooked according to package directions. Set aside

2. **Prepare Vegetables:**
   - Slice bell peppers, snap peas, and carrots into thin strips or bite-sized pieces.

3. **Sauté Ginger and Garlic:**
   - Warm the olive oil in a wok or big skillet over medium-high heat. Sauté minced ginger and garlic until fragrant.

4. **Stir-Fry Beef:**
   - Add thinly sliced beef strips to the pan. Cook until browned on all sides.

5. **Add Vegetables:**
   - Toss in mixed vegetables (bell peppers, snap peas, carrots). Stir-fry until vegetables are crisp-tender.

6. **Soy Sauce and Sesame Oil:**
   - Pour soy sauce and a drizzle of sesame oil over the beef and vegetables. Toss to coat evenly.

7. **Combine with Brown Rice:**
   - Add the cooked brown rice to the stir-fry. Mix until everything is well combined.

8. **Garnish with Green Onions:**
   - Garnish the stir-fry with sliced green onions for freshness and flavor.

9. **Serve Hot:**
   - Serve the Beef and Vegetable Stir-Fry immediately, providing a delicious and balanced high carb meal.

Nutritional Value (Approx. per Serving):

Calories: 450
Protein: 30g
Fat: 18g
Carbohydrates: 40g

Feel free to experiment with additional vegetables or adjust the seasoning to your liking. This stir-fry offers a delightful combination of lean beef, vibrant vegetables, and wholesome brown rice for a satisfying high carb dinner.

Salmon and Quinoa Bowl

Ingredients:
- Baked or grilled salmon fillets
- Quinoa, cooked
- Roasted Brussels sprouts
- Cherry tomatoes, halved
- Avocado, sliced
- Lemon wedges
- Olive oil
- Salt and pepper to taste

Instructions:

1. **Cook Quinoa:**
   - Cook quinoa according to package instructions. Set aside.

2. **Prepare Salmon:**
   - Bake or grill salmon fillets until they are cooked to your liking. Season with salt and pepper.

3. **Roast Brussels Sprouts:**
   - Roast Brussels sprouts in the oven with a drizzle of olive oil, salt, and pepper until they are caramelized and tender.

4. **Assemble the Bowl:**
   - In individual bowls, layer cooked quinoa as the base.

5. **Add Brussels Sprouts and Cherry Tomatoes:**
   - Place roasted Brussels sprouts and halved cherry tomatoes on top of the quinoa.

6. **Top with Salmon:**
   - Add the baked or grilled salmon fillets to the bowl.

7. **Sliced Avocado:**
   - Arrange sliced avocado over the salmon.

8. **Drizzle with Olive Oil:**
   - Drizzle a bit of olive oil over the bowl for added richness.

9. **Lemon Wedges:**
   - Serve with lemon wedges on the side for a citrusy touch.

10. **Season and Enjoy:**

   - Season the Salmon and Quinoa Bowl with salt
and pepper to taste. Enjoy this nutrient-rich and
satisfying high carb dinner!

Nutritional Value (Approx. per Serving):

Calories: 500
Protein: 35g
Fat: 25g
Carbohydrates: 35g

Feel free to customize this bowl with your favorite
vegetables or a drizzle of your preferred dressing.
This bowl combines the omega-3 richness of
salmon with the protein-packed quinoa and a
variety of colorful vegetables for a well-rounded and
flavorful meal.

Turkey and Vegetable Skillet

Ingredients:
- Ground turkey
- Sweet potatoes, diced
- Bell peppers, diced
- Black beans, drained and rinsed
- Taco seasoning
- Olive oil
- Avocado, sliced

- Greek yogurt (optional)

Instructions:

1. **Cook Ground Turkey:**
   - Over medium heat, preheat the olive oil in a pan. Cook the ground turkey until it begins to brown.

2. **Add Diced Sweet Potatoes:**
   - Add the diced sweet potatoes to the skillet. Cook until they are slightly softened.

3. **Include Bell Peppers:**
   - Stir in diced bell peppers and continue cooking until the vegetables are tender.

4. **Season with Taco Seasoning:**
   - Sprinkle taco seasoning over the turkey and vegetable mixture. Stir to coat evenly.

5. **Introduce Black Beans:**
   - Add drained and rinsed black beans to the skillet. Cook until everything is heated through.

6. **Serve Hot:**
   - Serve the Turkey and Vegetable Skillet hot, either as is or over a bed of cooked brown rice or quinoa.

7. **Top with Avocado:**

- Garnish the skillet with sliced avocado for creaminess and freshness.

8. **Optional Greek Yogurt:**
- If desired, add a dollop of Greek yogurt on top for extra richness.

9. **Season to Taste:**
- Season to taste with salt and pepper.

10. **Enjoy:**
- Enjoy this delicious and protein-packed Turkey and Vegetable Skillet as a flavorful high carb dinner.

Nutritional Value (Approx. per Serving):

Calories: 380
Protein: 30g
Fat: 15g
Carbohydrates: 30g

Feel free to customize the recipe by adding your favorite toppings like shredded cheese, salsa, or cilantro. This skillet provides a wholesome combination of lean protein from turkey, nutrient-dense sweet potatoes, and a variety of colorful vegetables for a satisfying and nutritious meal.

Vegetarian Chickpea Curry

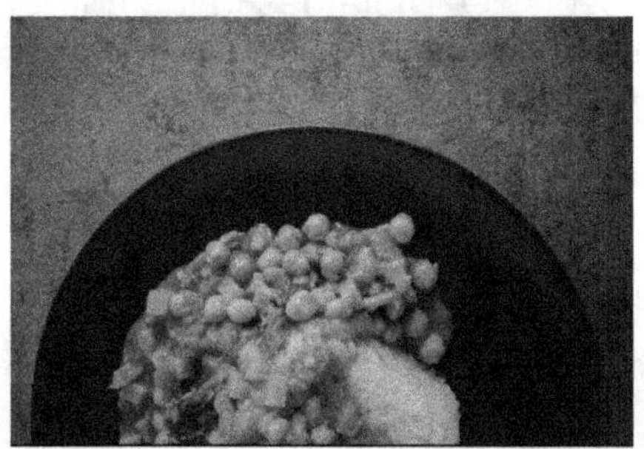

Ingredients:
- Chickpeas, cooked
- Coconut milk
- Sweet potatoes, diced
- Spinach
- Curry powder
- Onion, diced
- Garlic, minced
- Ginger, grated
- Basmati rice

Instructions:

1. **Cook Basmati Rice:**
   - Cook basmati rice per package directions. Set aside.

2. **Sauté Onion, Garlic, and Ginger:**
   - In a pot, sauté diced onion, minced garlic, and grated ginger until the onion becomes translucent.

3. **Add Sweet Potatoes:**
   - Add diced sweet potatoes to the pot. Cook until they start to soften.

4. **Stir in Curry Powder:**
   - Stir in curry powder, coating the sweet potatoes, onions, garlic, and ginger.

5. **Add Chickpeas:**
   - Add cooked chickpeas to the pot. Stir well to combine with the other ingredients.

6. **Pour Coconut Milk:**
   - Pour in coconut milk, ensuring it covers the chickpeas and sweet potatoes. Bring the mixture to a simmer.

7. **Simmer Until Sweet Potatoes are Tender:**
   - Let the curry simmer until the sweet potatoes are tender and the flavors meld together.

8. **Add Spinach:**
   - Stir in fresh spinach until it wilts into the curry.

9. **Season to Taste:**
   - Season the vegetarian chickpea curry with salt and pepper to taste.

10. **Serve Over Basmati Rice:**
    - Serve the Vegetarian Chickpea Curry over basmati rice, providing a delicious and hearty high carb dinner option.

Nutritional Value (Approx. per Serving):

Calories: 420
Protein: 15g
Fat: 20g
Carbohydrates: 50g

Feel free to garnish with chopped cilantro, a squeeze of lime juice, or a dollop of Greek yogurt for added freshness and flavor. This curry is a rich and satisfying blend of chickpeas, sweet potatoes, and spinach, offering a burst of Indian-inspired flavors.

Feel free to modify these recipes to suit your tastes and dietary requirements. Enjoy your high carb dinners!

SNACKS

Certainly! Here are three high-carb snack recipes with detailed instructions:

Banana and Almond Butter Toast

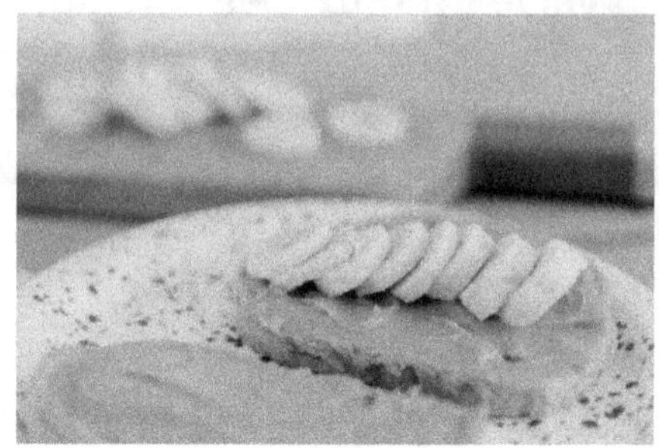

Ingredients:
- Whole grain bread
- Ripe bananas, sliced
- Almond butter

Instructions:

1. **Toast the Bread:**
   - Toast whole grain bread slices till crispy and golden.

2. **Spread Almond Butter:**
   - Spread a generous layer of almond butter on each slice of toasted bread.

3. **Arrange Banana Slices:**
   - Arrange slices of ripe banana on top of the almond butter.

4. **Optional Honey Drizzle:**
   - For added sweetness, drizzle a small amount of honey over the banana slices (optional).

5. **Serve:**
   - Enjoy your Banana and Almond Butter Toast as
a satisfying high-carb snack that combines complex
carbohydrates, healthy fats, and natural sweetness.

Nutritional Value (Approx. per Serving):

Calories: 300
Protein: 8g
Fat: 15g
Carbohydrates: 40g

This Banana and Almond Butter Toast is a simple
and nutritious high-carb snack or breakfast option.
Packed with healthy fats, natural sugars, and a
variety of textures, it's a delicious and energizing
choice. Customize with additional toppings like nuts
or seeds based on your preferences. Enjoy this
quick and satisfying toast!

Greek Yogurt Parfait

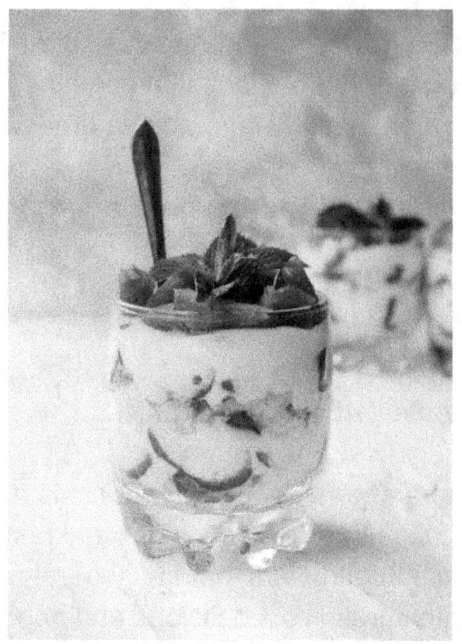

Ingredients:
- Greek yogurt
- Granola
- Mixed berries (strawberries, blueberries, raspberries)
- Honey

Instructions:

1. **Layer Greek Yogurt:**
   - In a serving glass or bowl, start by layering Greek yogurt at the bottom.

2. **Add Granola:**
   - Sprinkle a layer of granola over the Greek yogurt for added crunch and complex carbohydrates.

3. **Add Mixed Berries:**
   - Add a layer of mixed berries (strawberries, blueberries, raspberries) on top of the granola.

4. **Repeat Layers:**
   - Repeat the layers until the glass or bowl is filled, ending with a topping of mixed berries.

5. **Drizzle with Honey:**
   - Drizzle honey over the top for sweetness.

6. **Serve:**
   - Enjoy your Greek Yogurt Parfait as a delicious and nutrient-rich high-carb snack that provides a mix of protein, complex carbs, and antioxidants.

Nutritional Value (Approx. per Serving):

Calories: 350
Protein: 15g
Fat: 10g
Carbohydrates: 50g

This Greek Yogurt Parfait is a delicious and nutritious high-carb snack or breakfast option. Packed with protein, fiber, and a variety of textures, it's a satisfying and wholesome choice. Customize with your favorite fruits, granola, and toppings. Enjoy this refreshing and delightful parfait!

Sweet Potato Chips

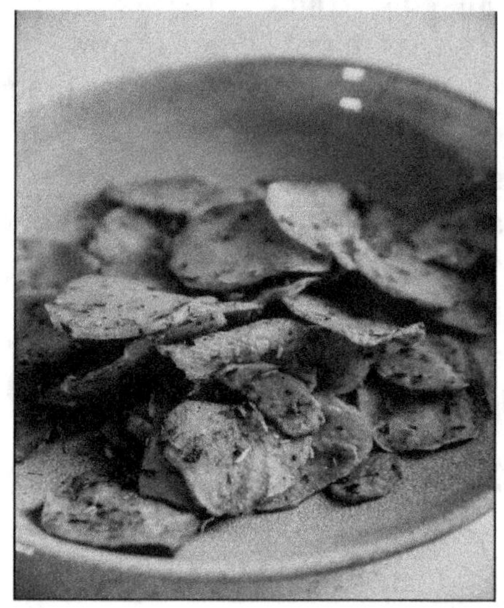

Ingredients:
- Sweet potatoes
- Olive oil
- Sea salt
- Paprika (optional)

Instructions:

1. **Preheat Oven:**
   - Set the oven temperature to 375°F, or 190°C.

2. **Slice Sweet Potatoes:**

- Thinly slice sweet potatoes into uniform rounds using a mandoline or a sharp knife.

3. **Coat with Olive Oil:**
- In a bowl, toss the sweet potato slices with olive oil until they are evenly coated.

4. **Season with Sea Salt (and Paprika):**
- Sprinkle sea salt over the sweet potato slices. For a hint of spice, add paprika as well.

5. **Arrange on Baking Sheet:**
- Spread out the spiced sweet potato slices on a baking pan in a single layer.

6. **Bake Until Crispy:**
- Bake in the preheated oven for approximately 15-20 minutes or until the sweet potato chips are crispy and golden brown.

7. **Cool and Serve:**
- Allow the sweet potato chips to cool before serving. They can be enjoyed as a crunchy, high-carb snack with a touch of natural sweetness.

Nutritional Value (Approx. per Serving):

Calories: 120
Protein: 2g
Fat: 5g
Carbohydrates: 18g

These Baked Sweet Potato Chips are a healthier alternative to traditional potato chips. Packed with vitamins and fiber, they make for a delicious and crunchy high-carb snack. Experiment with seasonings to suit your taste preferences. Enjoy these homemade chips guilt-free!

Feel free to modify these snacks to suit your tastes and dietary requirements. These options offer a combination of complex carbohydrates, healthy fats, and protein for a well-rounded snack experience.

DESSERTS

Certainly! Here are two delicious high-carb desserts with detailed instructions:

Fruit and Yogurt Parfait

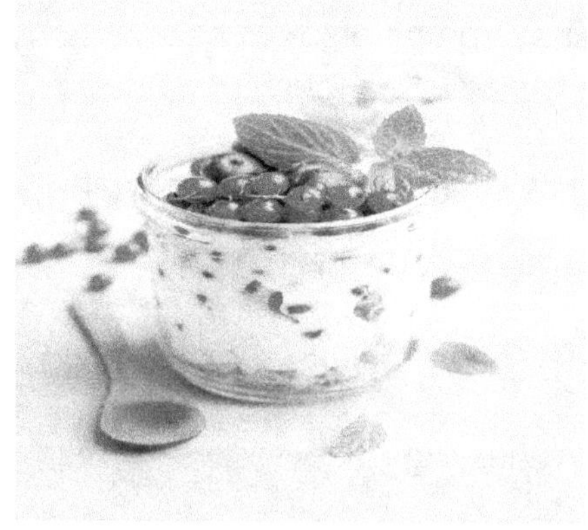

Ingredients:
- Greek yogurt
- Mixed berries (strawberries, blueberries, raspberries)
- Granola
- Honey

Instructions:

1. **Layer Greek Yogurt:**
   - In a serving glass or bowl, start by layering Greek yogurt at the bottom.

2. **Add Mixed Berries:**
   - Add a layer of mixed berries (strawberries, blueberries, raspberries) on top of the Greek yogurt.

3. **Sprinkle Granola:**
   - Sprinkle a layer of granola over the mixed berries for added texture and complex carbohydrates.

4. **Repeat Layers:**
   - Repeat the layers until the glass or bowl is filled, ending with a topping of mixed berries.

5. **Drizzle with Honey:**
   - Drizzle honey over the top for sweetness.

6. **Serve:**

- Enjoy your Fruit and Yogurt Parfait as a refreshing and high-carb dessert that combines the natural sweetness of fruits with the creaminess of Greek yogurt.

Nutritional Value (Approx. per Serving):

Calories: 300
Protein: 15g
Fat: 8g
Carbohydrates: 45g

This Fruit and Yogurt Parfait is a delightful and nutritious high-carb desserts.Packed with protein, fiber, and a burst of fruity flavors, it's a satisfying and refreshing choice. Customize with your favorite fruits and granola. Enjoy this simple and delicious parfait!

Rice Pudding

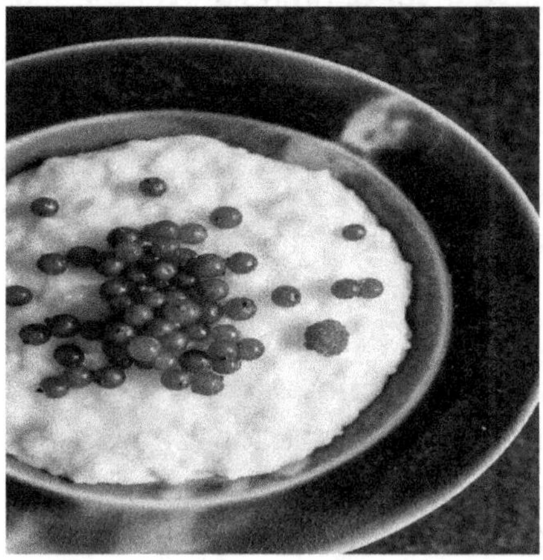

Ingredients:
- Cooked white rice
- Milk
- Sugar
- Vanilla extract
- Cinnamon
- Raisins (optional)

Instructions:

1. **Combine Rice and Milk:**
   - In a saucepan, combine cooked white rice and milk over medium heat.

2. **Stir in Sugar:**
   - Stir in sugar to sweeten the mixture to your liking.

3. **Add Vanilla Extract:**
   - Add a splash of vanilla extract for flavor.

4. **Simmer and Stir:**
   - To avoid sticking, let the mixture simmer while stirring often.

5. **Include Raisins (Optional):**
   - If desired, add raisins to the rice pudding for extra sweetness and texture.

6. **Sprinkle with Cinnamon:**

- Once the rice pudding has thickened to your preference, remove it from the heat and sprinkle with cinnamon.

7. **Serve Warm or Chilled:**
   - You can serve the rice pudding warm or cold, as you choose. It's a comforting and high-carb dessert option.

Nutritional Value (Approx. per Serving):

Calories: 250
Protein: 6g
Fat: 4g
Carbohydrates: 50g

This Classic Rice Pudding is a comforting and classic high-carb dessert. The creamy texture and subtle sweetness make it a timeless favorite. Customize by adding your favorite toppings like cinnamon, nutmeg, or a dollop of whipped cream. Enjoy this delicious and satisfying treat!

Feel free to adjust these recipes based on your taste preferences and dietary needs. These desserts offer a mix of complex carbohydrates, natural sugars, and satisfying flavors for your high-carb indulgence.

CHAPTER FIVE

RECIPES FOR LOW CARB DAYS

BREAKFAST

Certainly! Here are six low-carb breakfast recipes with detailed instructions:

Avocado and Egg Breakfast Bowl

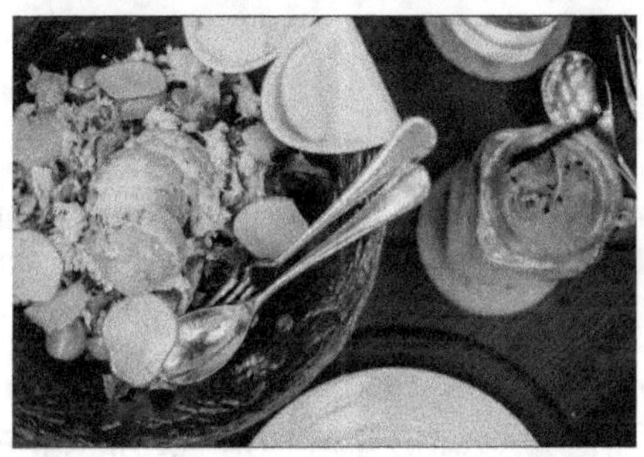

Ingredients:
- Ripe avocado, halved and pitted
- Eggs
- Salt and pepper
- Optional toppings: cherry tomatoes, feta cheese, hot sauce

Instructions:

1. **Preheat Oven:**

- Set the oven temperature to 425°F (220°C).

2. **Prepare Avocado Halves:**
   - Scoop out a small portion of the avocado flesh to create a well for the egg.

3. **Crack Eggs:**
   - Carefully crack an egg into each avocado half.

4. **Season and Bake:**
   - Sprinkle with salt and pepper. Place the avocado halves on a baking sheet and bake for about 12-15 minutes or until the eggs are cooked to your liking.

5. **Add Toppings:**
   - Optionally, top with cherry tomatoes, crumbled feta cheese, or a dash of hot sauce.

6. **Serve:**
   - Serve the Avocado and Egg Breakfast Bowl immediately for a nutritious and low-carb start to your day.

Nutritional Value (Approx. per Serving):

Calories: 300
Protein: 12g
Fat: 25g
Carbohydrates: 12g (Net carbs after deducting fiber)

This simple and delicious breakfast combines the creaminess of ripe avocado with the protein-packed goodness of baked eggs. Customize it with your favorite toppings for added flavor and enjoy a nutritious low-carb breakfast.

Spinach and Feta Omelette

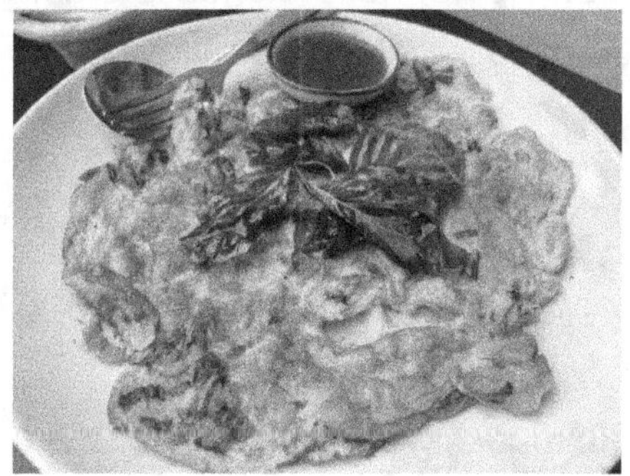

Ingredients:
- Eggs
- Fresh spinach
- Feta cheese, crumbled
- Salt and pepper
- Olive oil

Instructions:

1. **Whisk Eggs:**
   - Whisk the eggs together thoroughly in a bowl.

2. **Sauté Spinach:**

- In a non-stick skillet, heat olive oil and sauté fresh spinach until wilted.

3. **Pour Whisked Eggs:**
- Pour the whisked eggs over the sautéed spinach.

4. **Add Feta Cheese:**
- Evenly distribute the feta cheese crumbles over the eggs.

5. **Season and Fold:**
- Season with salt and pepper. Once the edges start to set, fold the omelette in half.

6. **Cook Through and Serve:**
- Continue cooking until the omelette is set. Place it on a platter and serve hot.

Nutritional Value (Approx. per Serving):

Calories: 250
Protein: 18g
Fat: 18g
Carbohydrates: 3g

This Spinach and Feta Omelette is a quick, easy, and nutritious breakfast option. The combination of spinach and feta adds a flavorful twist to classic eggs, making it a satisfying low-carb start to your day. Customize with additional herbs or veggies to suit your taste preferences. Enjoy!

Smoked Salmon and Cream Cheese Roll-Ups

Ingredients:
- Smoked salmon slices
- Cream cheese
- Cucumber, thinly sliced

Instructions:

1. **Spread Cream Cheese:**
   - Lay out smoked salmon slices and spread a thin layer of cream cheese over each slice.

2. **Add Cucumber Slices:**
   - Place thinly sliced cucumber over the cream cheese.

3. **Roll-Up:**
   - Each salmon slice should be tightly rolled.

4. **Slice and Serve:**
   - Slice the rolls into bite-sized pieces and serve as a flavorful and low-carb breakfast option.

Nutritional Value (Approx. per Serving):

Calories: 120
Protein: 10g

Fat: 8g
Carbohydrates: 2g

These Smoked Salmon and Cream Cheese Roll-Ups are not only delicious but also provide a balance of protein, healthy fats, and a refreshing crunch from the cucumber. Enjoy this elegant and satisfying low-carb dish!

Greek Yogurt Parfait with Berries

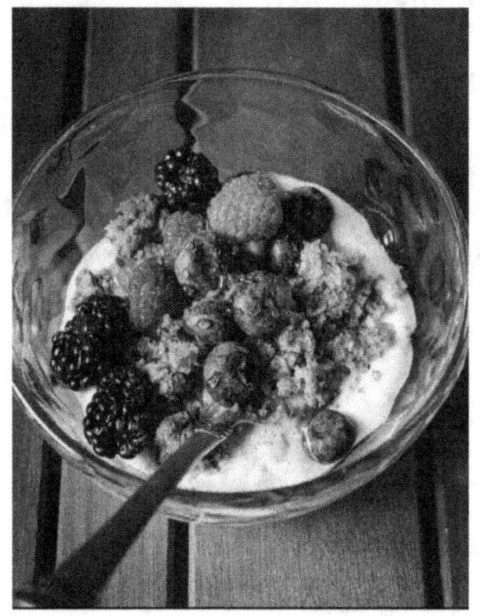

Ingredients:
- Greek yogurt
- Mixed berries (strawberries, blueberries, raspberries)

- Nuts (almonds, walnuts)
- Chia seeds (optional)
- Honey (optional)

Instructions:

1. **Layer Greek Yogurt:**
   - Place a layer of Greek yogurt in the bottom of a glass or bowl.

2. **Add Berries and Nuts:**
   - Add a layer of mixed berries and sprinkle with nuts.

3. **Repeat Layers:**
   - Layers should be repeated until the glass or bowl is full.

4. **Sprinkle Chia Seeds and Drizzle Honey (Optional):**
   - Optionally, sprinkle chia seeds over the top and drizzle with honey for added sweetness.

5. **Serve:**
   - Serve the Greek Yogurt Parfait chilled for a refreshing and low-carb breakfast.

Nutritional Value (Approx. per Serving):

Calories: 200
Protein: 15g
Fat: 8g

Carbohydrates: 15g (Net carbs after deducting fiber)

This Greek Yogurt Parfait with Berries is a delightful combination of creamy yogurt, vibrant berries, and crunchy nuts. Customize the layers based on your preferences, and enjoy a nutritious and satisfying low-carb option.

Cauliflower Hash Browns

Ingredients:
- Cauliflower, grated
- Eggs
- Almond flour
- Cheddar cheese, shredded
- Salt and pepper
- Olive oil

Instructions:

1. **Grate Cauliflower:**
   - Grate cauliflower using a box grater or food processor.

2. **Combine Ingredients:**
   - In a bowl, mix grated cauliflower, eggs, almond flour, shredded cheddar cheese, salt, and pepper.

3. **Form Patties:**

- Form the mixture into patties.

4. **Pan-Fry:**
   - Heat the olive oil in a pan over medium heat. Pan-fry the cauliflower patties until golden brown on each side.

5. **Serve Warm:**
   - Serve the Cauliflower Hash Browns warm for a delicious and low-carb alternative to traditional hash browns.

Nutritional Value (Approx. per Serving):

Calories: 120
Protein: 5g
Fat: 8g
Carbohydrates: 6g (Net carbs after deducting fiber)

These Cauliflower Hash Browns are a tasty and nutritious way to enjoy a low-carb breakfast. The combination of cauliflower, eggs, and cheese creates a satisfying texture, and they can be served with your favorite dipping sauce or alongside other breakfast items. Enjoy!

Keto Chia Seed Pudding

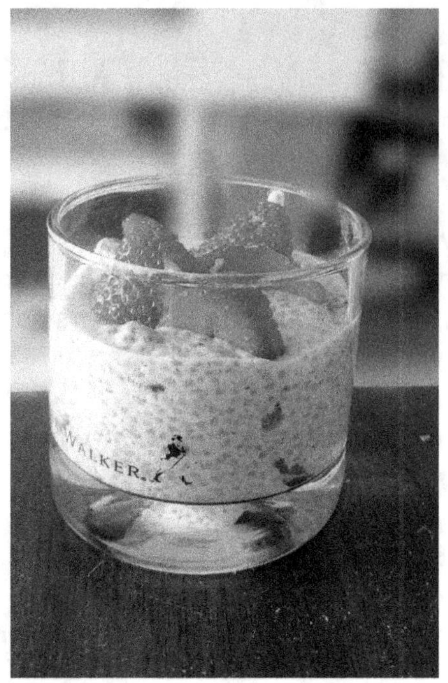

Ingredients:
- Chia seeds
- Unsweetened almond milk or coconut milk
- Vanilla extract
- Erythritol or stevia (optional)
- Berries for topping

Instructions:

1. **Mix Chia Seeds and Milk:**

- In a bowl or jar, mix chia seeds, unsweetened almond milk or coconut milk, vanilla extract, and sweetener if desired.

2. **Stir Well and Refrigerate:**
   - Stir well to combine, then refrigerate for at least 2-3 hours or overnight until the chia seeds absorb the liquid and form a pudding-like consistency.

3. **Top with Berries:**
   - Before serving, top the chia seed pudding with fresh berries.

4. **Serve Cold:**
   - Serve the Keto Chia Seed Pudding cold for a satisfying and low-carb breakfast option.

Nutritional Value (Approx. per Serving):

Calories: 150
Protein: 5g
Fat: 10g
Carbohydrates: 10g (Net carbs after deducting fiber)

This Keto Chia Seed Pudding is rich in fiber and healthy fats, making it a great option for those following a low-carb or ketogenic diet. Customize the sweetness and toppings based on your preferences, and enjoy a delicious and guilt-free treat!

Feel free to customize these recipes based on your taste preferences and dietary needs. These low-carb breakfast ideas offer a variety of flavors and textures to keep your mornings delicious and satisfying.

LUNCH

Certainly! Here are five low-carb lunch recipes with detailed instructions and approximate nutritional values per serving:

Grilled Chicken Salad

Ingredients:
- Chicken breast, boneless and skinless
- Mixed salad greens (lettuce, spinach, arugula)
- Cherry tomatoes, halved
- Cucumber, sliced
- Red onion, thinly sliced
- Avocado, sliced
- Olive oil
- Balsamic vinegar
- Dijon mustard
- Garlic, minced
- Salt and pepper

Instructions:

1. **Grill the Chicken:**
   - Add salt, pepper, and a little olive oil to the chicken breast to season it. Grill until fully cooked, with nice grill marks. Allow it to rest before slicing.

2. **Prepare Salad Greens:**
   - In a large bowl, combine mixed salad greens, halved cherry tomatoes, sliced cucumber, thinly sliced red onion, and sliced avocado.

3. **Make the Dressing:**
   - In a small bowl, whisk together olive oil, balsamic vinegar, Dijon mustard, minced garlic, salt, and pepper to create a vinaigrette.

4. **Slice the Chicken:**
   - Thinly slice the grilled chicken breast

5. **Assemble the Salad:**
   - Arrange the sliced chicken over the salad greens and vegetables.

6. **Drizzle with Dressing:**
   - Drizzle the vinaigrette over the salad, ensuring even distribution.

7. **Toss Gently:**
   - Gently toss the salad to evenly distribute the dressing among the components.

8. **Serve:**

  - Serve the Grilled Chicken Salad immediately as a delicious and nutritious low-carb meal.

Nutritional Value (Approx.):
- Calories: 400
- Protein: 30g
- Fat: 25g
- Carbohydrates: 15g

This Grilled Chicken Salad is not only low in carbs but also rich in protein and a variety of fresh vegetables, providing a satisfying and healthy option for lunch or dinner. Enjoy!

Zucchini Noodles with Pesto and Grilled Shrimp

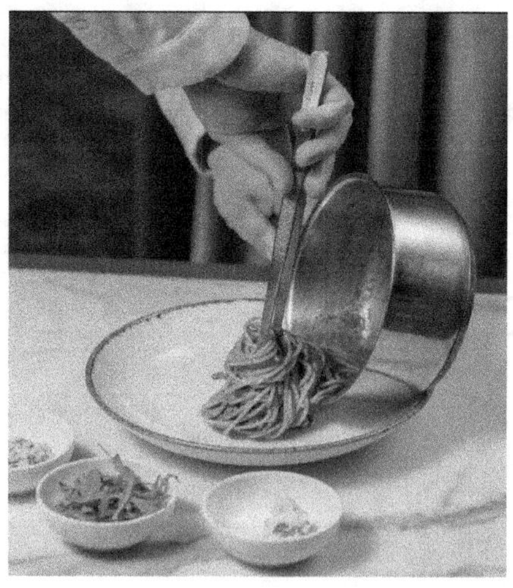

Ingredients:
- Zucchini, spiralized into noodles
- Grilled shrimp
- Pesto sauce (made with basil, pine nuts, Parmesan, olive oil)
- Cherry tomatoes, halved

Instructions:

1. **Prepare Zucchini Noodles:**
   - Spiralize the zucchini into noodles using a spiralizer.

2. **Grill Shrimp:**
   - Grill the shrimp until they are fully cooked. You can season them with salt, pepper, and a hint of olive oil.

3. **Make Pesto Sauce:**
   - In a food processor, combine fresh basil, pine nuts, grated Parmesan cheese, garlic, and olive oil. Blend until you achieve a smooth pesto sauce.

4. **Sauté Zucchini Noodles:**
   - In a pan over medium heat, sauté the zucchini noodles for a few minutes until they are just tender. Be careful not to overcook, as they should maintain a slight crunch.

5. **Combine Zoodles, Pesto, and Shrimp:**
   - Toss the sautéed zucchini noodles with the pesto sauce until well coated.

6. **Add Grilled Shrimp:**
   - Gently fold in the grilled shrimp, ensuring they are evenly distributed throughout the noodles.

7. **Top with Cherry Tomatoes:**
   - Garnish the dish with halved cherry tomatoes for a burst of freshness.

8. **Serve Warm:**
   - Serve the Zucchini Noodles with Pesto and Grilled Shrimp warm, and optionally, sprinkle some additional Parmesan cheese on top.

Nutritional Value (Approx.):
- Calories: 350
- Protein: 25g
- Fat: 20g
- Carbohydrates: 10g

This low-carb dish offers a delightful combination of zucchini noodles, flavorful pesto, and succulent grilled shrimp. It's not only delicious but also a great option for those looking for a lighter meal without sacrificing taste. Enjoy!

Cauliflower Fried Rice with Vegetables and Tofu

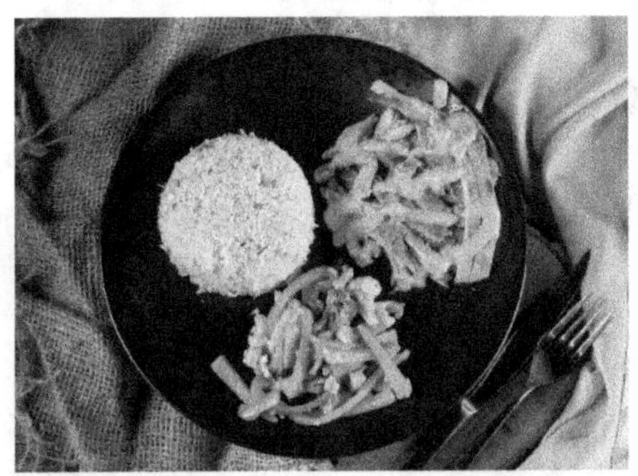

Ingredients:
- Cauliflower, grated (or cauliflower rice)
- Extra-firm tofu, pressed and cubed
- Mixed vegetables (carrots, peas, corn, broccoli), diced
- Scallions, chopped
- Garlic, minced
- Ginger, grated
- Soy sauce (low-sodium)
- Sesame oil
- Eggs, beaten (optional)
- Olive oil
- Salt and pepper to taste

Instructions:

1. **Prepare Cauliflower Rice:**
   - Grate the cauliflower using a box grater or food processor, or use pre-made cauliflower rice.

2. **Press and Cube Tofu:**

- Press the tofu to remove excess moisture, then cube it into bite-sized pieces.

3. **Sauté Tofu:**

- Heat the olive oil in a big pan or wok over medium-high heat. Sauté cubed tofu until golden brown on all sides. Take out of the pan and place aside.

4. **Sauté Vegetables:**

- If necessary, add a little extra oil to the same pan. Sauté mixed vegetables, minced garlic, and grated ginger until vegetables are tender-crisp.

5. **Add Cauliflower Rice:**

- Push the vegetables to the side of the pan and add the grated cauliflower. Sauté for a few minutes until the cauliflower is cooked but still has a bit of bite.

6. **Combine Tofu and Scallions:**

- Return the sautéed tofu to the pan. Add chopped scallions and mix everything together.

7. **Season with Soy Sauce and Sesame Oil:**

- Over the cauliflower rice mixture, drizzle some sesame oil and soy sauce. Toss well to coat evenly.

8. **Optional: Add Beaten Eggs:**

- Push the cauliflower rice mixture to one side of the pan, pour beaten eggs into the other side, and

scramble. Once cooked, mix the eggs with the rest
of the ingredients.

9. **Season to Taste:**
   - Season to taste with salt and pepper. If
necessary, adjust the soy sauce or sesame oil.

10. **Serve Warm:**
   - Serve the Cauliflower Fried Rice with
Vegetables and Tofu warm, garnished with
additional scallions if desired.

Nutritional Value (Approx.):
- Calories: 300
- Protein: 18g
- Fat: 15g
- Carbohydrates: 15g

This low-carb alternative to traditional fried rice is
packed with vegetables, tofu, and the delicious
flavors of soy sauce and sesame oil. It's a satisfying
and healthy dish for those seeking a lighter option.
Enjoy!

Turkey and Vegetable Lettuce Wraps

Ingredients:
- Ground turkey
- Lettuce leaves (butter lettuce works well)

- Bell peppers, diced
- Onion, diced
- Garlic, minced
- Avocado, sliced
- Greek yogurt (optional, for topping)
- Olive oil
- Ground cumin
- Chili powder
- Paprika
- Salt and pepper to taste

Instructions:

1. **Cook Ground Turkey:**
   - Heat the olive oil in a pan over medium heat. Add diced onion and garlic, sauté until softened. Once added, sauté the ground turkey until browned.

2. **Season with Spices:**
   - Sprinkle ground cumin, chili powder, paprika, salt, and pepper over the turkey mixture. Stir well to combine, allowing the spices to infuse.

3. **Add Bell Peppers:**
   - Add diced bell peppers to the skillet and cook until they are tender-crisp.

4. **Assemble Lettuce Wraps:**
   - Spoon the seasoned turkey and vegetable mixture onto individual lettuce leaves, creating wraps.

5. **Top with Avocado:**
   - Add slices of avocado on top of the turkey mixture in each lettuce wrap.

6. **Optional: Greek Yogurt Topping:**
   - Optionally, add a dollop of Greek yogurt on each wrap for a creamy element.

7. **Serve Warm:**
   - Serve the Turkey and Vegetable Lettuce Wraps warm. Roll them up and enjoy!

Nutritional Value (Approx.):
- Calories: 280
- Protein: 20g
- Fat: 15g
- Carbohydrates: 10g

These lettuce wraps provide a delicious and low-carb alternative to traditional wraps, offering a balance of lean protein, vibrant vegetables, and healthy fats from avocado. Customize the spices and toppings to suit your taste preferences. Enjoy this light and flavorful meal!

Salmon and Asparagus Foil Packets

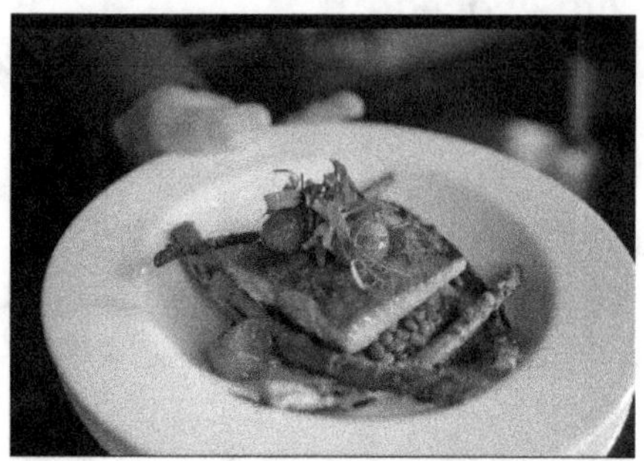

Ingredients:
- Salmon fillets
- Fresh asparagus spears
- Lemon slices
- Olive oil
- Garlic, minced
- Dill, chopped
- Salt and pepper to taste

Instructions:

1. **Preheat Oven:**
   - Preheat your oven to 400°F (200°C).

2. **Prepare Foil Packets:**
   - Cut sheets of aluminum foil. In the middle of each foil sheet, place a salmon fillet.

3. **Add Asparagus:**
   - Arrange fresh asparagus spears around the salmon fillets on each foil packet.

4. **Drizzle with Olive Oil:**
   - Drizzle olive oil over the salmon and asparagus. Ensure each fillet is coated.

5. **Season with Garlic, Dill, Salt, and Pepper:**
   - Sprinkle minced garlic and chopped dill over the salmon and asparagus. Season to taste with salt and pepper.

6. **Top with Lemon Slices:**
   - Place lemon slices on top of each salmon fillet for added freshness.

7. **Fold and Seal Packets:**
   - To make sealed packages, fold the foil over the salmon and asparagus. Ensure they are well-sealed to trap the flavors.

8. **Bake in the Oven:**
   - Place the foil packets on a baking sheet and bake in the preheated oven for approximately 15-20 minutes or until the salmon is cooked through and flakes easily.

9. **Serve Warm:**
   - Lift the foil packages with caution, then carefully place the asparagus and salmon onto plates. Serve warm.

Nutritional Value (Approx.):

- Calories: 350
- Protein: 30g
- Fat: 20g
- Carbohydrates: 5g

This simple and flavorful dish preserves the natural juices and aromas of salmon and asparagus. The foil packets make for easy cleanup, and the combination of garlic, dill, and lemon enhances the freshness of the ingredients. Enjoy this healthy and low-carb meal!

Please note that these nutritional values are approximate and can vary based on specific ingredients and portion sizes. Adjust quantities based on your dietary preferences and needs.

DINNER

Certainly! Here are five low-carb dinner recipes with detailed instructions and approximate nutritional values per serving:

Baked Lemon Herb Chicken

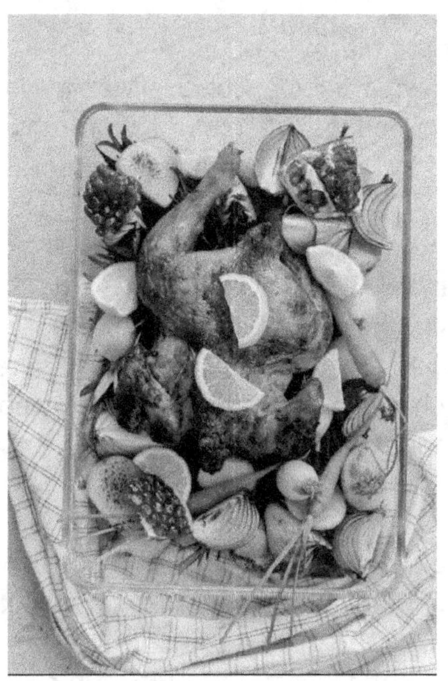

Ingredients:
- Chicken breasts
- Lemon juice
- Olive oil
- Garlic, minced
- Fresh herbs (rosemary, thyme, parsley)
- Salt and pepper

Instructions:

1. **Preheat Oven:**

- Set the oven temperature to 375°F, or 190°C.

2. **Prepare Marinade:**
   - In a bowl, mix lemon juice, olive oil, minced garlic, chopped fresh herbs (rosemary, thyme, parsley), salt, and pepper. Adjust quantities to taste.

3. **Marinate Chicken:**
   - Transfer the chicken breasts to a shallow dish or a plastic bag that can be sealed. Make sure every piece of chicken is thoroughly coated by pouring the marinade over it. Marinate for at least 30 minutes to allow flavors to infuse.

4. **Bake Chicken:**
   - Transfer the marinated chicken to a baking dish. Bake for 25 to 30 minutes, or until the internal temperature reaches 165°F (74°C), in a preheated oven.

5. **Baste with Juices:**
   - Occasionally, baste the chicken with the juices from the bottom of the baking dish to keep it moist.

6. **Broil for Crispy Top (Optional):**
   - If you desire a crispy top, you can broil the chicken for the last 2-3 minutes, keeping a close eye to prevent burning.

7. **Check Doneness:**

- Ensure the chicken is fully cooked, with no pink in the center.

8. **Rest Before Serving:**
   - Allow the baked lemon herb chicken to rest for a few minutes before slicing.

9. **Serve Warm:**
   - Serve the baked lemon herb chicken warm, garnished with additional fresh herbs if desired.

Nutritional Value (Approx.):
- Calories: 250
- Protein: 30g
- Fat: 12g
- Carbohydrates: 1g

This Baked Lemon Herb Chicken is a simple yet flavorful dish, making it a perfect option for a low-carb meal. The combination of zesty lemon, aromatic herbs, and succulent chicken creates a delicious and wholesome dinner. Enjoy!

Cauliflower and Broccoli Alfredo Bake

Ingredients:
- Cauliflower florets
- Broccoli florets
- Low-carb Alfredo sauce

- Mozzarella cheese, shredded
- Parmesan cheese, grated

Instructions:

1. **Steam Cauliflower and Broccoli:**
   - Steam cauliflower and broccoli florets until they are slightly tender. This can be done using a steamer or by boiling for a few minutes.

2. **Preheat Oven:**
   - Set the oven temperature to 375°F, or 190°C.

3. **Layer Vegetables in Baking Dish:**
   - In a baking dish, layer the steamed cauliflower and broccoli.

4. **Pour Alfredo Sauce:**
   - Pour a generous amount of low-carb Alfredo sauce over the cauliflower and broccoli, ensuring even coverage.

5. **Add Cheese:**
   - Sprinkle shredded mozzarella and grated Parmesan cheese over the top, creating a cheesy layer.

6. **Repeat Layers:**
   - Repeat the process, creating additional layers of vegetables, Alfredo sauce, and cheese until the baking dish is filled.

7. **Top with Cheese:**
   - Finally, add a layer of cheese on top.

8. **Bake in the Oven:**
   - Bake for 20-25 minutes, or until the cheese is melted and bubbling and the rims are golden brown, in a preheated oven.

9. **Broil for Crispy Top (Optional):**
   - If desired, you can broil the dish for an additional 2-3 minutes for a crispy and golden top. Keep a close eye to prevent burning.

10. **Serve Warm:**
   - Allow the Cauliflower and Broccoli Alfredo Bake to cool slightly before serving. Scoop out portions and serve warm.

****Nutritional Value (Approx.):****
- Calories: 180
- Protein: 12g
- Fat: 14g
- Carbohydrates: 5g

This low-carb bake offers a creamy and cheesy alternative to traditional Alfredo pasta dishes, with the added nutritional benefits of cauliflower and broccoli. It's a comforting and satisfying option for a flavorful dinner. Enjoy!

Grilled Salmon with Avocado Salsa

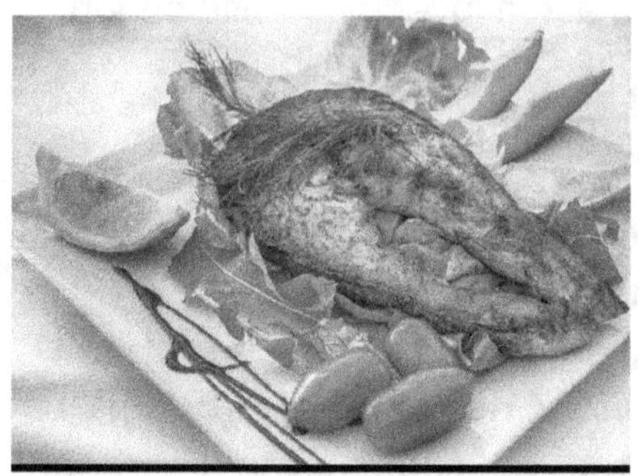

Ingredients:
- Salmon fillets
- Avocado, diced
- Cherry tomatoes, diced
- Red onion, finely chopped
- Cilantro, chopped
- Lime juice
- Olive oil
- Salt and pepper

Instructions:

1. **Preheat Grill:**
   - Preheat your grill to medium-high heat.

2. **Season Salmon:**
   - Season the salmon fillets with salt and pepper.

3. **Grill Salmon:**

- Grill the salmon fillets for 4-5 minutes per side or until the salmon is cooked to your liking. Internal temperature should be at 145°F (63°C).

4. **Prepare Avocado Salsa:**
   - In a bowl, combine diced avocado, cherry tomatoes, finely chopped red onion, chopped cilantro, lime juice, and a drizzle of olive oil. Gently mix to combine.

5. **Top Salmon with Salsa:**
   - Once the salmon is grilled, transfer it to a serving platter or individual plates. Spoon the avocado salsa generously over the grilled salmon fillets.

6. **Garnish and Serve:**
   - Garnish with additional cilantro and lime wedges if desired. Serve immediately while the salmon is warm.

****Nutritional Value (Approx.):****
- Calories: 300
- Protein: 25g
- Fat: 20g
- Carbohydrates: 10g

This Grilled Salmon with Avocado Salsa is a vibrant and flavorful low-carb dish. The combination of grilled salmon and the freshness of the avocado salsa creates a delightful contrast of textures and tastes. It's a nutritious and satisfying option for a healthy dinner. Enjoy!

Eggplant Lasagna

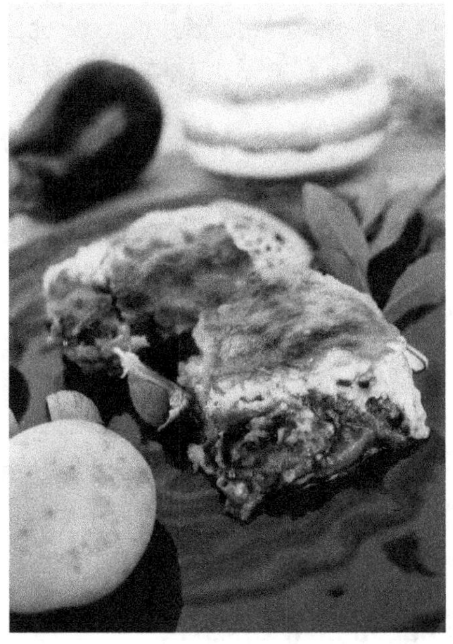

Ingredients:
- Eggplant, thinly sliced lengthwise
- Ground beef or turkey
- Low-carb marinara sauce
- Ricotta cheese
- Mozzarella cheese, shredded
- Parmesan cheese, grated
- Italian seasoning
- Olive oil

- Salt and pepper

Instructions:

1. **Preheat Oven:**
   - Set the oven temperature to 375°F, or 190°C.

2. **Brown Ground Meat:**
   - In a skillet, brown ground beef or turkey over medium-high heat. Season with salt and pepper.

3. **Prepare Eggplant:**
   - Thinly slice the eggplant lengthwise. If desired, sprinkle slices with salt and let them sit for 15 minutes to release excess moisture. Pat dry with a paper towel.

4. **Layer Eggplant and Meat:**
   - In a baking dish, layer the sliced eggplant and cooked ground meat.

5. **Add Marinara Sauce:**
   - Pour low-carb marinara sauce over the layers, ensuring even coverage.

6. **Dollop Ricotta:**
   - Add dollops of ricotta cheese over the sauce layer.

7. **Sprinkle Mozzarella and Parmesan:**
   - Over the ricotta layer, top with shredded mozzarella and grated Parmesan cheese.

8. **Repeat Layers:**
   - Repeat the layering process, finishing with a final layer of marinara sauce and a generous sprinkle of mozzarella and Parmesan.

9. **Season with Italian Seasoning:**
   - Sprinkle Italian seasoning over the top for added flavor.

10. **Bake in the Oven:**
    - Bake in the preheated oven for 30-35 minutes or until the cheese is melted and bubbly, and the eggplant is tender.

11. **Broil for Crispy Top (Optional):**
    - For a golden and crispy top, you can broil the Eggplant Lasagna for an additional 2-3 minutes. Keep a close eye to prevent burning.

12. **Rest Before Serving:**
    - Allow the lasagna to rest for a few minutes before slicing.

13. **Serve Warm:**
    - Serve the Eggplant Lasagna warm, and garnish with fresh herbs if desired.

Nutritional Value (Approx.):
- Calories: 280
- Protein: 20g
- Fat: 18g

- Carbohydrates: 10g

This low-carb Eggplant Lasagna is a flavorful and satisfying alternative to traditional lasagna, offering the richness of meat, cheese, and marinara without the pasta. It's a delicious and nutritious option for a comforting dinner. Enjoy!

Chicken and Vegetable Stir-Fry

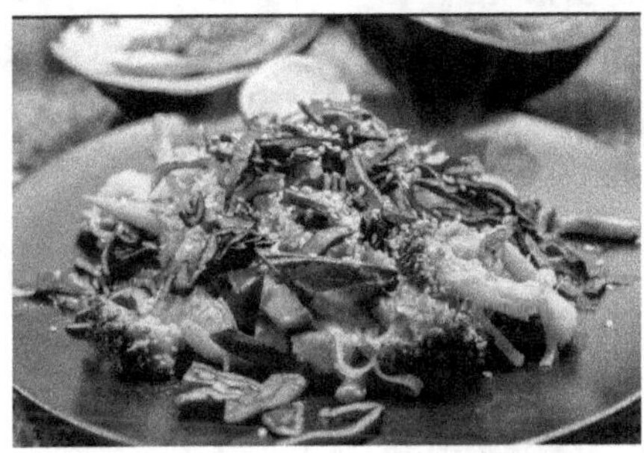

Ingredients:
- Chicken breast, thinly sliced
- Broccoli florets
- Bell peppers, sliced
- Zucchini, sliced
- Soy sauce (low-sodium)
- Sesame oil
- Garlic, minced
- Ginger, grated
- Olive oil
- Cauliflower rice

Instructions:

1. **Prep Ingredients:**
   - Thinly slice chicken breast, chop broccoli into florets, and slice bell peppers and zucchini.

2. **Heat Olive Oil:**
   - Warm the olive oil in a wok or big skillet over medium-high heat.

3. **Sauté Chicken:**
   - Add sliced chicken to the hot pan. Cook until browned and cooked through.

4. **Add Garlic and Ginger:**
   - Add minced garlic and grated ginger to the chicken. Sauté until fragrant.

5. **Stir in Vegetables:**
   - Add broccoli florets, sliced bell peppers, and zucchini to the wok. Stir-fry until vegetables are tender-crisp.

6. **Drizzle with Soy Sauce and Sesame Oil:**
   - Drizzle low-sodium soy sauce and sesame oil over the chicken and vegetables. Toss to coat evenly.

7. **Serve Over Cauliflower Rice:**
   - Over a bed of cauliflower rice, serve the stir-fried chicken and vegetables.

8. **Garnish and Enjoy:**
   - If desired, garnish with chopped green onions or sesame seeds. Serve immediately.

****Nutritional Value (Approx.):****
- Calories: 280
- Protein: 25g
- Fat: 14g
- Carbohydrates: 10g

This Chicken and Vegetable Stir-Fry is a quick and flavorful low-carb option, providing a colorful array of vegetables and lean protein. The use of cauliflower rice keeps the dish light and carb-conscious. Enjoy this delicious stir-fry as a healthy and satisfying meal!

Adjust ingredients and portion sizes to meet specific dietary requirements. Enjoy these flavorful and nutritious low-carb dinner options!

SNACKS

Certainly! Here are three low-carb snack recipes with detailed instructions and approximate nutritional values:

Cucumber and Cream Cheese Bites

Ingredients:
- Cucumber, sliced
- Cream cheese, softened
- Smoked salmon (optional)
- Fresh dill, chopped (for garnish)

Instructions:

1. **Slice the Cucumber:**
   - Slice the cucumber into rounds, creating a base for the cream cheese bites.

2. **Spread Cream Cheese:**
   - Spread a thin layer of softened cream cheese on each cucumber slice.

3. **Add Smoked Salmon (Optional):**
   - Optionally, top each cream cheese-covered cucumber slice with a small piece of smoked salmon.

4. **Garnish with Fresh Dill:**
   - Garnish the bites with chopped fresh dill for added flavor and a pop of color.

5. **Serve:**
   - Arrange the Cucumber and Cream Cheese Bites on a serving platter.

6. **Optional Variation:**
   - For a different twist, you can add a sprinkle of black pepper, a squeeze of lemon juice, or a pinch of red pepper flakes.

Nutritional Value (Approx. per Serving):
- Calories: 80
- Protein: 5g
- Fat: 6g
- Carbohydrates: 2g

These Cucumber and Cream Cheese Bites make for a refreshing and low-carb snack, perfect for a light and flavorful treat. Adjust the toppings and seasonings to suit your taste preferences. Enjoy!

Cheese and Almond Stuffed Jalapeños

Ingredients:
- Jalapeños, halved and seeds removed
- Cream cheese
- Shredded cheddar cheese
- Almonds, whole or chopped

Instructions:

1. **Preheat the Oven:**
   - Preheat the oven to 375°F (190°C).

2. **Prepare Jalapeños:**
   - Cut jalapeños in half lengthwise and remove the seeds to control the heat.

3. **Cheese Mixture:**
   - In a bowl, mix cream cheese and shredded cheddar cheese until well combined.

4. **Stuff Jalapeños:**
   - Stuff the cheese mixture into each half of a jalapeño. Use a spoon to press the cheese into the jalapeño.

5. **Add Almonds:**
   - Top each stuffed jalapeño with a whole or chopped almond, pressing it gently into the cheese.

6. **Bake:**
   - Place the stuffed jalapeños on a baking sheet and bake for 15-20 minutes or until the jalapeños are tender and the cheese is melted and slightly golden.

7. **Serve:**
   - Remove from the oven and let them cool slightly before serving.

8. **Optional Garnish:**
   - Garnish with fresh cilantro or serve with a side of sour cream for dipping.

Nutritional Value (Approx. per Serving):

- Calories: 120
- Protein: 5g
- Fat: 10g
- Carbohydrates: 3g

These Cheese and Almond Stuffed Jalapeños make a delicious and spicy low-carb appetizer or snack. The combination of creamy cheese, the crunch of almonds, and the heat of jalapeños creates a flavorful bite. Adjust the spice level by removing or keeping the jalapeño seeds. Enjoy responsibly!

Avocado and Tuna Lettuce Wraps

Ingredients:
- Romaine lettuce leaves
- Avocado, sliced
- Canned tuna, drained
- Olive oil
- Lemon juice
- Salt and pepper to taste

Instructions:

1. **Prepare Lettuce Wraps:**
   - Lay out Romaine lettuce leaves on a clean surface, creating a base for the wraps.

2. **Slice Avocado:**

- Slice the avocado into thin strips.

3. **Prepare Tuna Mixture:**
  - In a bowl, mix the drained canned tuna with a drizzle of olive oil, lemon juice, salt, and pepper. Adjust to taste.

4. **Assemble Wraps:**
  - Place a few slices of avocado on each lettuce leaf, and top with a portion of the tuna mixture.

5. **Fold and Serve:**
  - Fold the lettuce leaves around the avocado and tuna, creating wraps.

6. **Serve Immediately:**
  - Serve the Avocado and Tuna Lettuce Wraps immediately while they are fresh and flavorful.

Nutritional Value (Approx. per Serving):
- Calories: 200
- Protein: 15g
- Fat: 15g
- Carbohydrates: 5g

These Avocado and Tuna Lettuce Wraps provide a light and satisfying low-carb option. The creaminess of avocado complements the protein-rich tuna, creating a flavorful and nutritious snack or meal. Customize with additional herbs or spices for added flavor. Enjoy!

These low-carb snack options are not only delicious but also provide a good balance of nutrients for your low-carb day. Adjust the amounts to suit your food preferences and nutritional requirements. Enjoy!

DESSERTS

Certainly! Here are three low-carb dessert recipes with detailed instructions and approximate nutritional values:

Berries and Cream Parfait

Ingredients:
- Mixed berries (strawberries, blueberries, raspberries)
- Whipped cream (unsweetened)
- Stevia or erythritol (to taste)

Instructions:

1. **Prepare Berries:**
   - Wash and hull strawberries. If using larger berries, you can slice them for easier layering.

2. **Layer Berries:**

- In a glass or bowl, create the first layer by placing a portion of mixed berries at the bottom.

3. **Add Whipped Cream:**
   - Spoon a layer of unsweetened whipped cream over the berries.

4. **Repeat Layers:**
   - Repeat the process, layering berries and whipped cream until you reach the top of the glass or bowl.

5. **Sweeten to Taste:**
   - Sweeten the parfait with stevia or erythritol to taste. Adjust based on your preferred level of sweetness.

6. **Garnish:**
   - Garnish the top with a few whole berries for a visually appealing finish.

7. **Serve Chilled:**
   - Refrigerate the parfait for a short time if you'd like it chilled before serving.

8. **Enjoy:**
   - Serve the Berries and Cream Parfait as a delightful and low-carb dessert.

Nutritional Value (Approx. per Serving):
- Calories: 150
- Protein: 2g

- Fat: 12g
- Carbohydrates: 10g (Net carbs after deducting fiber)

This Berries and Cream Parfait offers a light and refreshing low-carb dessert option. The combination of vibrant mixed berries and unsweetened whipped cream provides a satisfying sweetness without compromising your carb goals. Adjust sweetness levels to suit your taste preferences. Enjoy!

Chocolate Avocado Mousse

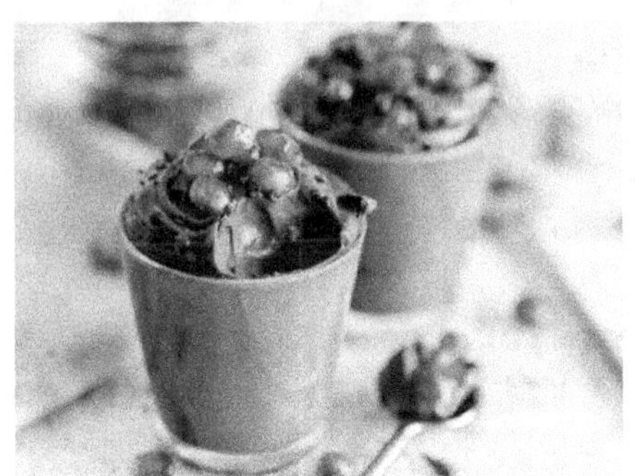

Ingredients:
- Ripe avocados
- Unsweetened cocoa powder
- Almond milk (unsweetened)
- Monk fruit sweetener or stevia (to taste)
- Vanilla extract

Instructions:

1. **Blend Avocado Mixture:**
   - In a blender, combine ripe avocados, unsweetened cocoa powder, almond milk, stevia or monk fruit sweetener, and vanilla extract.

2. **Blend Until Smooth:**
   - Blend until the mixture is smooth and creamy, ensuring that there are no avocado lumps.

3. **Adjust Sweetness:**
   - Taste the mousse and adjust the sweetness by adding more stevia or monk fruit sweetener if needed.

4. **Chill in Refrigerator:**
   - Transfer the chocolate avocado mixture to a bowl and refrigerate for at least an hour to allow it to chill and firm up.

5. **Serve in Cups or Bowls:**
   - Once chilled, portion the mousse into individual cups or bowls.

6. **Optional Garnish:**
   - Optionally, garnish the mousse with a sprinkle of cocoa powder for an extra touch of chocolate.

7. **Enjoy:**
   - Serve the Chocolate Avocado Mousse as a rich and creamy low-carb dessert.

Nutritional Value (Approx. per Serving):
- Calories: 180
- Protein: 3g
- Fat: 15g
- Carbohydrates: 8g (Net carbs after deducting
fiber)

This Chocolate Avocado Mousse is a decadent and
satisfying low-carb dessert that combines the
richness of chocolate with the creamy texture of
avocado. Adjust sweetness to your liking and enjoy
this guilt-free treat!

Chia Seed Pudding with Almond Milk

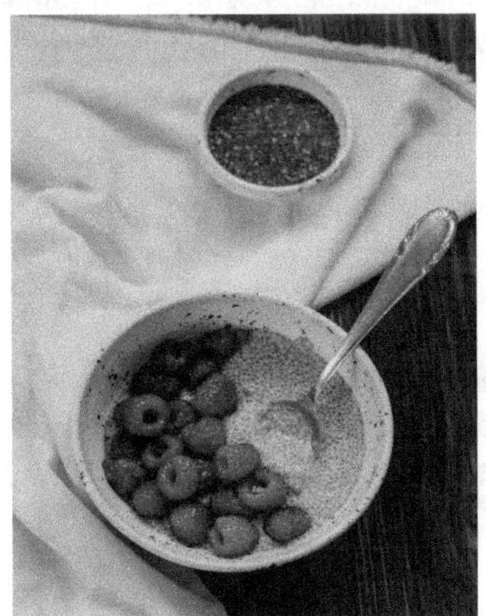

Ingredients:
- Chia seeds

- Almond milk (unsweetened)
- Vanilla extract
- Stevia or erythritol (to taste)
- Fresh berries for topping

Instructions:

1. **Combine Ingredients:**
   - In a bowl, mix chia seeds, almond milk, a splash of vanilla extract, and your preferred sweetener (stevia or erythritol). Make sure the chia seeds are dispersed evenly by giving it a good stir.

2. **Let it Sit:**
   - To keep the mixture from clumping, let it settle for a few minutes before stirring it once more. Refrigerate for at least 30 minutes or overnight, allowing the chia seeds to absorb the liquid and create a pudding-like consistency.

3. **Stir Before Serving:**
   - Before serving, give the chia pudding another good stir to ensure a smooth texture.

4. **Portion into Cups:**
   - Portion the chia seed pudding into individual cups or bowls.

5. **Top with Fresh Berries:**
   - Top the pudding with fresh berries for added flavor and texture.

6. **Serve Chilled:**
   - Serve the Chia Seed Pudding with Almond Milk chilled and enjoy.

****Nutritional Value (Approx. per Serving):****
- Calories: 120
- Protein: 4g
- Fat: 8g
- Carbohydrates: 10g (Net carbs after deducting fiber)

This Chia Seed Pudding with Almond Milk is a delightful low-carb dessert or snack. The chia seeds provide a dose of fiber and omega-3 fatty acids, while the almond milk adds a creamy texture. Customize with your favorite toppings or a sprinkle of cinnamon for extra flavor. Enjoy!

These low-carb desserts offer a sweet treat while keeping your carb intake in check. Adjust sweetness levels according to your preferences, and feel free to get creative with additional toppings or flavorings. Enjoy!

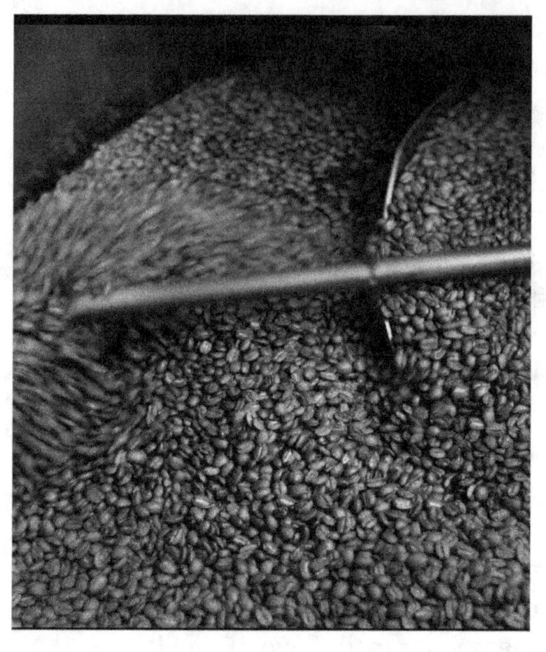

CHAPTER SIX

RECIPES FOR MODERATE CARB DAY

BREAKFAST

Certainly! Here are five moderate-carb breakfast recipes with detailed instructions and approximate nutritional values:

Classic Oatmeal with Berries

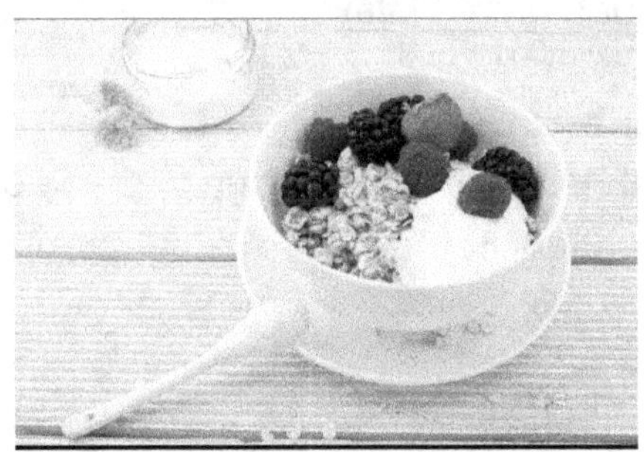

Ingredients:
- Rolled oats
- Milk (dairy or plant-based)
- Fresh berries (strawberries, blueberries)
- Honey or maple syrup for sweetness

Instructions:

1. **Cook Oatmeal:**
   - In a saucepan, cook rolled oats with your choice of milk according to the package instructions. Stir occasionally until the oats are soft and have absorbed the liquid.

2. **Prepare Berries:**
   - Wash and hull strawberries. If using larger berries, you can slice them for easier mixing.

3. **Top with Berries:**
   - Once the oatmeal is cooked, top it with a generous serving of fresh berries. Mix them into the oatmeal for a burst of flavor.

4. **Sweeten to Taste:**
   - Drizzle honey or maple syrup over the oatmeal to add sweetness. Adjust the sweetness to your liking.

5. **Serve Warm:**
   - Spoon the Classic Oatmeal with Berries into bowls and serve warm.

Nutritional Value (Approx. per Serving):
- Calories: 300
- Protein: 8g
- Fat: 5g
- Carbohydrates: 55g

This Classic Oatmeal with Berries provides a wholesome and nutritious breakfast, combining the heartiness of oats with the freshness of mixed berries. Customize the sweetness level to suit your taste, and enjoy a comforting start to your day!

Whole Grain Toast with Smashed Avocado

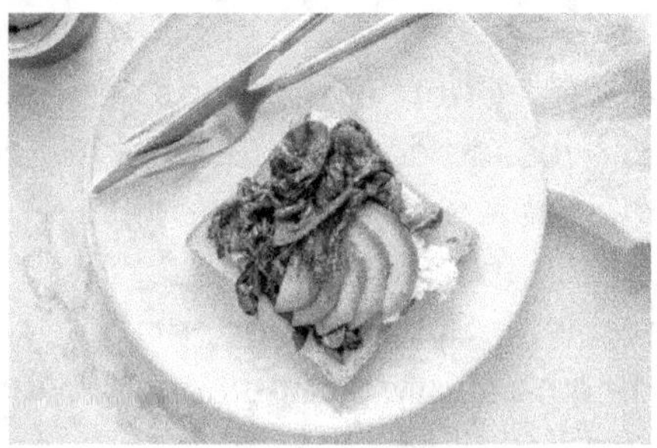

Ingredients:
- Whole grain bread slices, toasted
- Ripe avocado
- Cherry tomatoes, sliced
- Salt and pepper to taste

Instructions:

1. **Prepare Avocado:**
   - Cut a ripe avocado in half and remove the pit. Scoop the avocado flesh into a bowl.

2. **Smash Avocado:**

- Using a fork, smash the avocado until it reaches
your desired consistency.

3. **Toast Bread:**
   - Toast whole grain bread slices until they are
golden brown and crisp.

4. **Spread Avocado on Toast:**
   - Spread the smashed avocado evenly over the
toasted whole grain bread slices.

5. **Add Sliced Cherry Tomatoes:**
   - Top the avocado-covered toast with sliced
cherry tomatoes.

6. **Season with Salt and Pepper:**
   - Sprinkle a pinch of salt and pepper over the
tomatoes for added flavor.

7. **Serve:**
   - Serve the Whole Grain Toast with Smashed
Avocado as a delicious and nutritious breakfast.

Nutritional Value (Approx. per Serving):
- Calories: 250
- Protein: 8g
- Fat: 15g
- Carbohydrates: 25g

This Whole Grain Toast with Smashed Avocado is
a satisfying and nutrient-rich breakfast option. The
combination of whole grain bread, creamy avocado,

and juicy tomatoes provides a balance of flavors and textures. Customize with additional toppings or seasonings according to your preferences. Enjoy!

Greek Yogurt Parfait with Granola

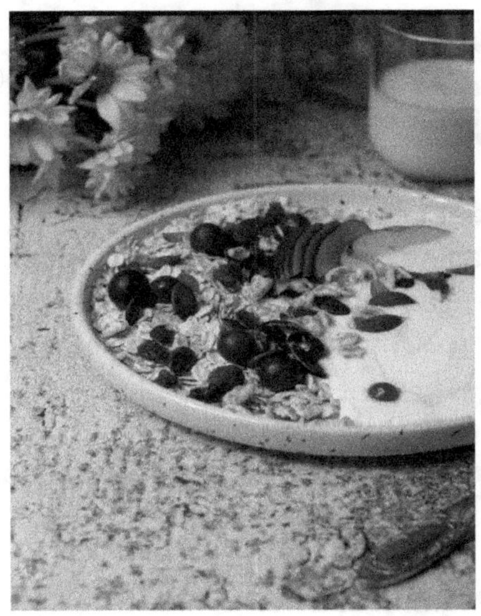

Ingredients:
- Greek yogurt (unsweetened)
- Granola (low-sugar)
- Mixed berries
- Chia seeds (optional)

Instructions:

1. **Layer Greek Yogurt:**

- In a glass or bowl, create the first layer by spooning a portion of unsweetened Greek yogurt.

2. **Add Granola Layer:**
   - Sprinkle a layer of low-sugar granola over the Greek yogurt.

3. **Include Mixed Berries:**
   - Add a layer of mixed berries on top of the granola.

4. **Repeat Layers:**
   - Repeat the layering process until you reach the top of the glass or bowl, ensuring an even distribution of ingredients.

5. **Optional Chia Seeds:**
   - Optionally, sprinkle chia seeds on top for added texture and nutritional benefits.

6. **Serve Immediately:**
   - Serve the Greek Yogurt Parfait with Granola immediately to maintain the crunch of the granola.

Nutritional Value (Approx. per Serving):
- Calories: 350
- Protein: 15g
- Fat: 10g
- Carbohydrates: 45g

This Greek Yogurt Parfait with Granola is a delightful and filling breakfast or snack. The combination of creamy Greek yogurt, crunchy granola, and fresh berries provides a satisfying balance of textures and flavors. Customize with your favorite berries and enjoy a nutritious start to your day!

Scrambled Eggs with Spinach and Feta

Ingredients:
- Eggs
- Fresh spinach
- Feta cheese, crumbled
- Salt and pepper to taste

Instructions:

1. **Scramble Eggs:**
   - Crack eggs into a bowl and beat them until well combined.

2. **Cook Spinach:**
   - In a pan over medium heat, add fresh spinach and cook until wilted.

3. **Add Eggs to Spinach:**
   - Over the cooked spinach, pour the beaten eggs.

4. **Scramble Together:**

- Stir the eggs and spinach together, allowing the eggs to cook through.

5. **Add Feta Cheese:**
   - Once the eggs are almost fully cooked, add crumbled feta cheese to the mixture.

6. **Season with Salt and Pepper:**
   - To taste, add salt and pepper to the scrambled eggs.

7. **Serve Warm:**
   - Continue cooking until the eggs are fully set but still moist. Serve the Scrambled Eggs with Spinach and Feta while warm.

Nutritional Value (Approx. per Serving):
- Calories: 280
- Protein: 18g
- Fat: 20g
- Carbohydrates: 5g

This Scrambled Eggs with Spinach and Feta is a protein-packed breakfast that combines the richness of eggs with the freshness of spinach and the savory flavor of feta cheese. It's a quick and delicious way to start your day with a nutritious meal. Adjust the quantities based on your preferences and dietary needs. Enjoy!

Whole Wheat Pancakes with Maple Syrup

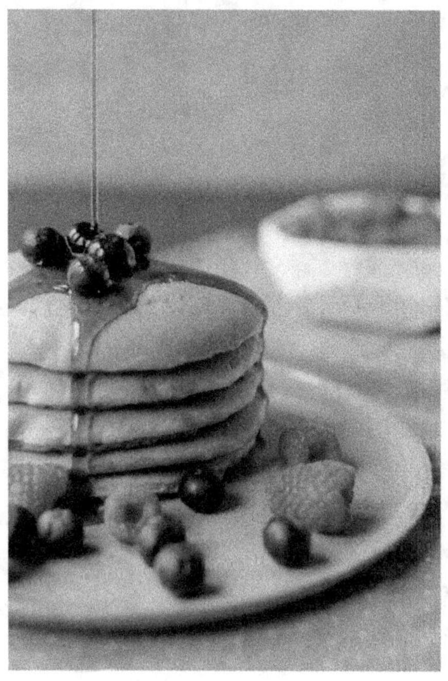

Ingredients:
- Whole wheat pancake mix
- Milk or water (per the directions on the package)
- Maple syrup for topping
- Sliced bananas (optional)

Instructions:

1. **Prepare Pancake Batter:**
   - Mix whole wheat pancake batter according to package instructions, using water or milk.

2. **Cook Pancakes:**
   - Cook pancakes on a griddle or skillet over medium heat until bubbles form on the surface, then flip and cook until golden brown.

3. **Stack Pancakes:**
   - Stack the cooked pancakes on a plate.

4. **Top with Maple Syrup:**
   - Drizzle maple syrup generously over the stack of pancakes.

5. **Optional Banana Topping:**
   - Optionally, top the pancakes with sliced bananas for added sweetness and flavor.

6. **Serve Warm:**
   - Serve the Whole Wheat Pancakes with Maple Syrup warm.

Nutritional Value (Approx. per Serving):
- Calories: 320
- Protein: 8g
- Fat: 5g
- Carbohydrates: 60g

These Whole Wheat Pancakes with Maple Syrup offer a wholesome and comforting breakfast. The use of whole wheat adds fiber and nutrients to your morning meal, while the maple syrup provides a delightful sweetness. Customize with your favorite toppings or fruits for additional flavor. Enjoy your delicious and nutritious pancake stack!

These moderate-carb breakfast recipes offer a balance of nutrients and flavors, providing a satisfying start to your day. Adjust portions based on your dietary preferences and nutritional needs. Enjoy!

LUNCH

Certainly! Here are four moderate-carb lunch recipes with detailed instructions and approximate nutritional values:

Chickpea and Avocado Wrap

Ingredients:
- Whole grain wrap
- Chickpeas, canned and drained
- Avocado, sliced
- Cherry tomatoes, sliced
- Spinach leaves
- Hummus for spreading

Instructions:

1. **Prepare Chickpeas:**

- Rinse and drain canned chickpeas. You can optionally mash them slightly for added texture.

2. **Spread Hummus:**
   - Lay the whole grain wrap on a clean surface and spread a layer of hummus evenly over the surface.

3. **Assemble Wrap:**
   - Place chickpeas, sliced avocado, cherry tomatoes, and spinach leaves along the center of the wrap.

4. **Fold and Roll:**
   - Fold in the sides of the wrap and then roll it up tightly from the bottom, creating a secure wrap.

5. **Slice and Serve:**
   - Slice the Chickpea and Avocado Wrap in half diagonally and serve.

Nutritional Value (Approx. per Serving):
- Calories: 350
- Protein: 12g
- Fat: 18g
- Carbohydrates: 40g

This Chickpea and Avocado Wrap is a delicious and nutrient-packed lunch option. The combination of chickpeas, creamy avocado, and fresh vegetables provides a satisfying and flavorful meal. Adjust ingredients and add your favorite spices or

sauces to personalize this wrap to your taste.
Enjoy!

Grilled Salmon Salad

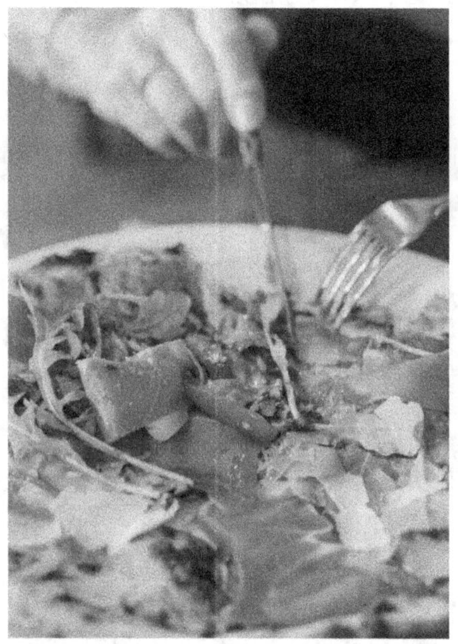

Ingredients:
- Grilled salmon fillet
- Mixed greens (spinach, arugula, kale)
- Cherry tomatoes, halved
- Red onion, thinly sliced
- Balsamic vinaigrette dressing

Instructions:

1. **Prepare Grilled Salmon:**
   - Grill the salmon fillet until it's fully cooked. Allow it to cool slightly before assembling the salad.

2. **Mix Greens:**
   - In a large bowl, combine mixed greens, such as spinach, arugula, and kale.

3. **Add Cherry Tomatoes and Red Onion:**
   - Toss in halved cherry tomatoes and thinly sliced red onion with the mixed greens.

4. **Flake Grilled Salmon:**
   - Flake the grilled salmon into bite-sized pieces and gently mix it with the greens and vegetables.

5. **Dressing:**
   - Dress the salad with the balsamic vinaigrette dressing. Toss until everything is evenly coated.

6. **Serve:**
   - Portion the Grilled Salmon Salad onto plates and serve immediately.

Nutritional Value (Approx. per Serving):
- Calories: 380
- Protein: 25g
- Fat: 22g
- Carbohydrates: 20g

This Grilled Salmon Salad is a light and flavorful option for a moderate-carb lunch. The combination of grilled salmon, fresh greens, and vibrant vegetables creates a well-balanced and nutritious meal. Customize with additional toppings or herbs according to your preferences. Enjoy the health benefits and deliciousness of this satisfying salad!

Mediterranean Turkey Pita Pocket

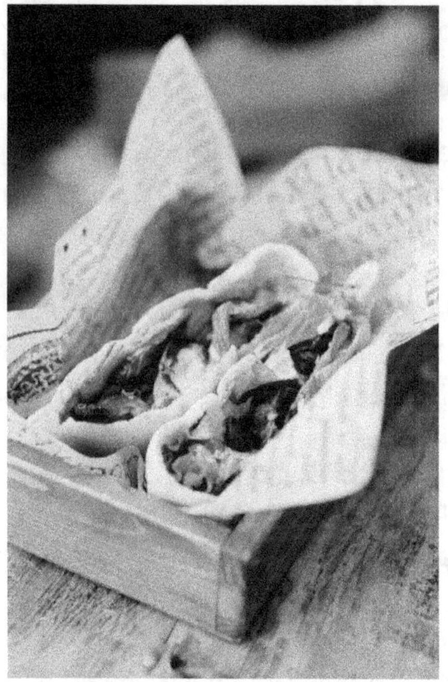

Ingredients:
- Whole wheat pita pockets
- Ground turkey, cooked
- Hummus
- Cucumber, diced

- Kalamata olives, sliced
- Tzatziki sauce for dressing

Instructions:

1. **Cook Ground Turkey:**
   - Cook ground turkey until fully cooked, breaking it into crumbles.

2. **Prepare Pita Pockets:**
   - Gently warm the whole wheat pita pockets.

3. **Spread Hummus:**
   - Fill each pita pocket with a generous amount of hummus.

4. **Fill with Turkey and Vegetables:**
   - Fill the pita pockets with the cooked ground turkey, diced cucumber, and sliced Kalamata olives.

5. **Drizzle with Tzatziki Sauce:**
   - Drizzle tzatziki sauce over the filling for a creamy and flavorful touch.

6. **Serve:**
   - Serve the Mediterranean Turkey Pita Pockets as a delicious and portable lunch.

Nutritional Value (Approx. per Serving):
- Calories: 320
- Protein: 22g
- Fat: 15g

- Carbohydrates: 25g

These Mediterranean Turkey Pita Pockets are a delightful combination of lean protein, fresh vegetables, and savory sauces. The whole wheat pita adds fiber, making it a satisfying and healthy lunch option. Customize with your favorite Mediterranean toppings for additional flavors. Enjoy this convenient and flavorful meal!

Caprese Quinoa Bowl

Ingredients:
- Cooked quinoa
- Fresh mozzarella balls
- Cherry tomatoes, halved
- Fresh basil leaves
- Balsamic glaze for drizzling

Instructions:

1. **Prepare Quinoa:**
   - As directed on the package, prepare the quinoa and allow it to cool.

2. **Assemble Bowl:**
   - In a bowl, layer cooked quinoa as the base.

3. **Add Mozzarella and Tomatoes:**

- Scatter fresh mozzarella balls and halved cherry tomatoes over the quinoa.

4. **Tear Basil Leaves:**
   - Tear fresh basil leaves and sprinkle them over the bowl.

5. **Drizzle with Balsamic Glaze:**
   - Finish by drizzling the entire bowl with balsamic glaze.

6. **Serve:**
   - Gently toss the ingredients in the bowl before serving to combine the flavors.

Nutritional Value (Approx. per Serving):
- Calories: 380
- Protein: 15g
- Fat: 20g
- Carbohydrates: 30g

This Caprese Quinoa Bowl offers a light and refreshing option for a moderate-carb lunch. The combination of quinoa, fresh mozzarella, tomatoes, and basil creates a Mediterranean-inspired dish. Drizzling with balsamic glaze enhances the flavors, making it a delicious and satisfying meal. Customize according to your preferences and enjoy this nutritious bowl!

These moderate-carb lunch recipes offer a balance of protein, healthy fats, and carbohydrates. Adjust portion sizes based on your nutritional needs and enjoy a satisfying and flavorful midday meal.

DINNER

Certainly! Here are five moderate-carb dinner recipes with detailed instructions and approximate nutritional values:

Grilled Chicken and Vegetable Skewers

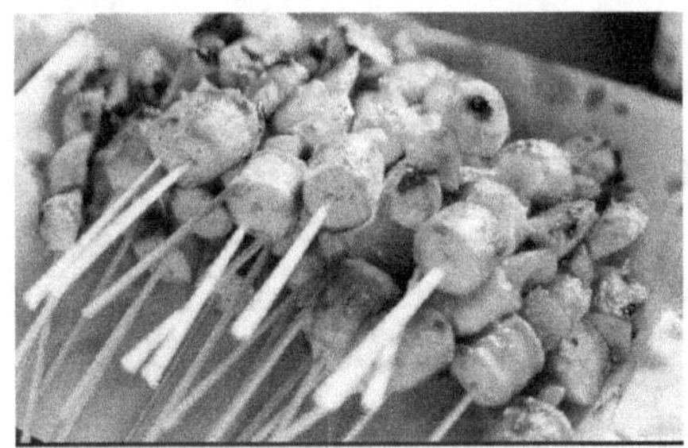

Ingredients:
- Chicken breast, cubed
- Bell peppers (assorted colors), sliced
- Zucchini, sliced
- Cherry tomatoes
- Olive oil
- Garlic, minced
- Mixed herbs (rosemary, thyme, oregano)
- Salt and pepper to taste

Instructions:

1. **Marinate Chicken:**
   - In a bowl, combine cubed chicken with olive oil, minced garlic, mixed herbs, salt, and pepper. Give it at least half an hour to marinate.

2. **Prepare Vegetables:**
   - Slice bell peppers, zucchini, and halve cherry tomatoes.

3. **Skewer Assembly:**
   - Thread marinated chicken, bell peppers, zucchini, and cherry tomatoes onto skewers, alternating for a colorful mix.

4. **Grill:**
   - Preheat the grill. Grill the skewers over medium-high heat, turning occasionally, until chicken is fully cooked and vegetables are charred and tender.

5. **Serve:**
   - Transfer the Grilled Chicken and Vegetable Skewers to a serving plate. Optionally, sprinkle extra herbs and serve with your favorite dipping sauce.

Nutritional Value (Approx. per Serving):
- Calories: 400
- Protein: 30g

- Fat: 15g
- Carbohydrates: 35g

These Grilled Chicken and Vegetable Skewers offer a delightful combination of tender, flavorful chicken and colorful, grilled vegetables. Perfect for a moderate-carb dinner, this dish is not only delicious but also a visually appealing addition to your meal. Adjust ingredients and seasoning to suit your taste preferences. Enjoy!

Shrimp and Broccoli Stir-Fry

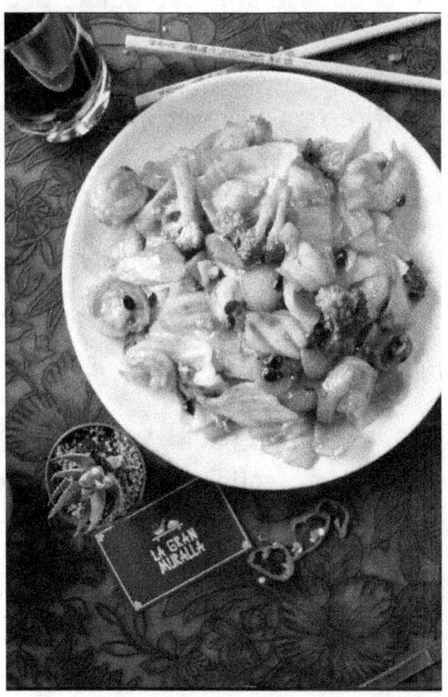

Ingredients:
- Shrimp, peeled and deveined
- Broccoli florets
- Soy sauce
- Fresh ginger, minced
- Garlic, minced
- Sesame oil
- Brown rice (cooked)

Instructions:

1. **Stir-Fry Shrimp and Broccoli:**
   - In a wok or large skillet, heat sesame oil over medium-high heat. Add minced ginger and garlic, stir briefly, then add shrimp and broccoli.

2. **Cook Shrimp and Broccoli:**
   - Stir-fry until shrimp turn pink and opaque, and broccoli is crisp-tender.

3. **Soy Sauce Seasoning:**
   - Pour soy sauce over the shrimp and broccoli. Continue stirring to coat evenly.

4. **Serve Over Brown Rice:**
   - Serve the Shrimp and Broccoli Stir-Fry over cooked brown rice.

Nutritional Value (Approx. per Serving):
- Calories: 380
- Protein: 25g
- Fat: 10g

- Carbohydrates: 45g

This Shrimp and Broccoli Stir-Fry is a quick and flavorful option for a moderate-carb dinner. Packed with protein and vibrant vegetables, it's a healthy and satisfying meal. Adjust the level of soy sauce and sesame oil according to your taste preferences. Enjoy this delicious stir-fry over a bed of nutritious brown rice!

Turkey and Vegetable Quinoa Bowl

Ingredients:
- Ground turkey
- Quinoa (cooked)
- Mixed vegetables (carrots, peas, corn)
- Olive oil
- Onion, finely chopped
- Garlic, minced
- Italian herbs (oregano, basil, thyme)
- Salt and pepper to taste

Instructions:

1. **Cook Ground Turkey:**
   - Heat the olive oil in a pan over medium heat. Add finely chopped onion and minced garlic. Sauté until softened.

2. **Brown Turkey:**

- Add ground turkey to the skillet and cook until browned, breaking it into crumbles.

3. **Add Mixed Vegetables:**
   - Stir in mixed vegetables (carrots, peas, corn) and cook until they are tender.

4. **Season with Herbs:**
   - Sprinkle Italian herbs over the turkey and vegetable mixture. Add salt and pepper to taste. Stir to combine.

5. **Combine with Quinoa:**
   - Mix the cooked quinoa into the turkey and vegetable mixture, ensuring everything is well incorporated.

6. **Serve:**
   - Portion the Turkey and Vegetable Quinoa Bowl into serving dishes.

Nutritional Value (Approx. per Serving):
- Calories: 420
- Protein: 30g
- Fat: 15g
- Carbohydrates: 40g

This Turkey and Vegetable Quinoa Bowl is a well-balanced and nutritious dinner option. Packed with lean protein, colorful vegetables, and quinoa, it provides a satisfying and flavorful meal. Customize the vegetable mix and seasonings to suit your taste preferences. Enjoy this delicious and wholesome bowl!

Salmon and Asparagus Bake

Ingredients:
- Salmon fillets
- Fresh asparagus spears
- Lemon slices
- Garlic cloves, minced
- Olive oil
- Dill, dried or fresh
- Salt and pepper to taste
- Brown rice or quinoa (optional, for serving)

Instructions:

1. **Preheat Oven:**
   - Preheat your oven to 400°F (200°C).

2. **Prepare Salmon and Asparagus:**
   - Place salmon fillets and fresh asparagus spears on a baking sheet lined with parchment paper.

3. **Seasoning:**
   - Drizzle olive oil over the salmon and asparagus. Sprinkle minced garlic, dill, salt, and pepper evenly. Place lemon slices on top for added flavor.

4. **Bake:**

   - Bake for 15 to 20 minutes in a preheated oven,
or until the salmon is cooked through and flake
easily with a fork.

5. **Serve:**
   - Serve the Salmon and Asparagus Bake over
brown rice or quinoa if desired.

Nutritional Value (Approx. per Serving):
- Calories: 380
- Protein: 30g
- Fat: 20g
- Carbohydrates: 25g

This Salmon and Asparagus Bake is a simple and
healthy dinner option. The combination of salmon's
omega-3 fatty acids and the nutritious asparagus
makes for a flavorful and well-balanced meal.
Serve it over brown rice or quinoa for an extra dose
of fiber. Enjoy this delicious and nourishing dish!

Vegetarian Stuffed Bell Peppers

Ingredients:
- Bell peppers, halved and seeds removed
- Quinoa (cooked)
- Black beans, drained and rinsed
- Corn kernels
- Diced tomatoes
- Mexican blend cheese

- Taco seasoning
- Fresh cilantro, chopped
- Salt and pepper to taste
- Avocado (optional, for topping)

Instructions:

1. **Prepare Bell Peppers:**
   - Cut bell peppers in half, removing seeds and membranes. Preheat the oven to 375°F (190°C).

2. **Quinoa Mixture:**
   - In a bowl, mix cooked quinoa, black beans, corn, diced tomatoes, taco seasoning, chopped cilantro, salt, and pepper.

3. **Stuff Bell Peppers:**
   - Spoon the quinoa mixture into each bell pepper half, pressing down gently. Top each with a sprinkle of Mexican blend cheese.

4. **Bake:**
   - Place the stuffed bell peppers on a baking dish. Bake in the preheated oven for 25-30 minutes or until the peppers are tender.

5. **Optional Toppings:**
   - Garnish with additional chopped cilantro and serve with slices of avocado if desired.

Nutritional Value (Approx. per Serving):
- Calories: 350

- Protein: 15g
- Fat: 15g
- Carbohydrates: 40g

These Vegetarian Stuffed Bell Peppers are a colorful and satisfying dish. Packed with protein, fiber, and a variety of vegetables, they make a nutritious and flavorful meal. Customize the stuffing with your favorite ingredients and enjoy a delicious, meatless option for dinner!

These moderate-carb dinner recipes provide a variety of flavors and nutrients. Adjust portion sizes based on your dietary needs, and enjoy these delicious and balanced meals!

SNACKS

Certainly! Here are two snack recipes for a moderate-carb day, along with detailed instructions and approximate nutritional values:

Apple slices with a small handful of almonds

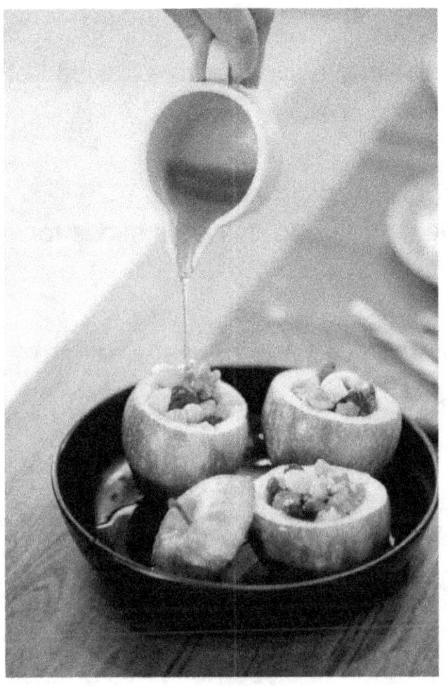

Ingredients:
- Apple, sliced
- Almonds, a small handful

Instructions:

1. **Slice the Apple:**
   - Wash and slice the apple into thin, bite-sized pieces.

2. **Prepare Almonds:**
   - Take a small handful of almonds.

3. **Combine:**
   - Enjoy the apple slices with a handful of almonds
for a balanced snack.

4. **Optional Additions:**
   - Sprinkle cinnamon on apple slices for extra
flavor.

Nutritional Value (Approx. per Serving):
- Calories: 150
- Protein: 4g
- Fat: 8g
- Carbohydrates: 18g

This simple and nutritious snack of apple slices with
almonds provides a combination of fiber, healthy
fats, and a touch of sweetness. It's a quick and
satisfying option for a moderate-carb snack that
can keep you energized throughout the day. Enjoy
this wholesome and delicious treat!

CHAPTER SEVEN

NUTRITIONAL TIPS AND TRICKS

The following are some nutrition tips and tricks to put in to considerations:

1. **Balanced Meals:**
A balanced meal includes a combination of carbohydrates, proteins, and healthy fats. Carbs provide energy, proteins support muscle health, and fats aid in nutrient absorption. This combination helps maintain steady energy levels throughout the day.

2. **Portion Control:**
Portion control involves being mindful of the amount of food you eat. Using smaller plates, measuring portions, and paying attention to hunger cues can prevent overeating, supporting weight management and digestion.

3. **Hydration:**
Staying hydrated is crucial for overall health. Water supports digestion, nutrient transport, and temperature regulation. Drinking water before meals can also help control appetite, preventing overconsumption.

4. **Whole Foods:**

Whole foods are high in fiber and other minerals. Fruits, vegetables, whole grains, lean proteins, and healthy fats provide a wide range of vitamins and minerals, promoting overall health and reducing the risk of chronic diseases.

5. **Meal Planning:**
Planning meals in advance allows for balanced and varied nutrition. It helps avoid relying on convenient but often less nutritious options. Meal planning can also save time and reduce the likelihood of unhealthy impulse choices.

6. **Snack Smart:**
Nutrient-dense snacks, such as fruits, nuts, and yogurt, can curb hunger between meals. Avoiding highly processed snacks high in sugars and unhealthy fats supports sustained energy and overall health.

7. **Mindful Eating:**
Being totally present throughout meals is what mindful eating entails. By paying attention to flavors, textures, and hunger cues, individuals can enjoy food more, recognize fullness, and make healthier choices.

8. **Read Labels:**
Reading food labels helps identify hidden sugars, sodium, and unhealthy fats in processed foods. Choosing products with minimal additives supports a more wholesome diet.

9. **Cook at Home:**
   Cooking at home provides control over ingredients and cooking methods. It allows for the creation of healthier meals using fresh, whole ingredients, and promotes a greater awareness of what goes into your food.

10. **Limit Added Sugars:**
   Excessive added sugars can contribute to various health issues. Choosing natural sources of sweetness, like fruits, and limiting processed foods helps control sugar intake and supports better overall health.

11. **Include Fiber:**
   Fiber aids in digestion, helps maintain a healthy weight, and stabilizes blood sugar levels. Foods rich in fiber, such as whole grains, legumes, and vegetables, contribute to a well-rounded and satisfying diet.

12. **Protein Intake:**
   Protein is essential for muscle repair, immune function, and satiety. Including a variety of protein sources, such as lean meats, dairy, and plant-based options, ensures adequate intake for overall health.

13. **Limit Processed Foods:**
   Highly processed meals are frequently high in unhealthy chemicals, preservatives, and salt.

Reducing the consumption of these foods supports better nutritional intake and overall well-being.

14. **Moderation:**
Enjoying treats in moderation rather than complete restriction promotes a healthy relationship with food. It allows for occasional indulgences while maintaining a balanced and sustainable diet.

15. **Consult a Professional:**
Seeking advice from a registered dietitian or nutritionist provides personalized guidance based on individual needs and goals. Professional advice can help navigate dietary challenges, address specific health concerns, and create a tailored nutrition plan.

SUPPLEMENTS RECOMMENDATIONS

1. **Multivitamin:**
- **Purpose:** To fill potential nutrient gaps and ensure overall vitamin and mineral intake.
- **Considerations:** Choose a high-quality multivitamin with essential vitamins and minerals.

2. **Omega-3 Fatty Acids:**
- **Purpose:** Supports heart health, brain function, and reduces inflammation.

- **Considerations:** Fish oil or algae-based supplements are rich in omega-3s. Consult with a healthcare professional for appropriate dosage.

3. **Vitamin D:**
   - **Purpose:** Essential for bone health, immune function, and overall well-being.
   - **Considerations:** Especially important for individuals with limited sun exposure. Check blood levels and consult with a healthcare provider for proper dosage.

4. **Calcium:**
   - **Purpose:** Supports bone health, muscle function, and nerve transmission.
   - **Considerations:** Adequate calcium intake is crucial, especially for those with low dairy consumption. Consider combining with vitamin D for optimal absorption.

5. **Iron:**
   - **Purpose:** Important for oxygen transport and preventing iron-deficiency anemia.
   - **Considerations:** Consult with a healthcare professional to determine the need for supplementation, as excessive iron can be harmful.

6. **Probiotics:**
   - **Purpose:** Supports gut health and a balanced microbiome.

- **Considerations:** Choose a probiotic with diverse strains. It can be beneficial for digestive issues and immune function.

7. **Magnesium:**
   - **Purpose:** Supports muscle and nerve function, energy production, and bone health.
   - **Considerations:** Individuals with low dietary magnesium intake may benefit from supplementation. Consult with a healthcare professional for appropriate dosage.

8. **B Vitamins (B12, B6, Folate):**
   - **Purpose:** Essential for energy metabolism, nerve function, and DNA synthesis.
   - **Considerations:** Particularly important for vegetarians/vegans (B12) and pregnant women (folate). Ensure a balanced B-complex supplement or targeted B-vitamin as needed.

9. **Vitamin C:**
   - **Purpose:** Supports the immune system, skin health, and acts as an antioxidant.
   - **Considerations:** Can be obtained through diet, but supplementation may be considered during times of increased immune stress.

10. **Zinc:**
    - **Purpose:** Supports immune function, wound healing, and DNA synthesis.

  - **Considerations:** Important for those with zinc deficiency or during periods of increased need. Consult with a healthcare professional.

11. **Creatine:**
  - **Purpose:** Aids in muscle strength and power, especially for those engaged in high-intensity exercise.
  - **Considerations:** Generally safe and well-tolerated. Consult a healthcare expert, especially if you have any pre-existing health issues.

12. **Melatonin:**
  - **Purpose:** Regulates sleep-wake cycles and may help with sleep disturbances.
  - **Considerations:** Useful for individuals with insomnia or irregular sleep patterns. For proper usage, consult a healthcare practitioner.

Before beginning any new supplement regimen, always consult with a healthcare expert. Individual needs vary, and professional guidance ensures safe and effective supplementation based on specific health considerations.

HYDRATION IMPORTANCE

The following are the importance of hydration:

1. **Cellular Function:**

Water is essential for various cellular processes, including nutrient transport, chemical reactions, and overall cell function. Adequate hydration ensures cells can perform their functions optimally.

2. **Temperature Regulation:**
Sweating is the body's natural cooling mechanism. Proper hydration helps regulate body temperature, preventing overheating during physical activity or in hot environments.

3. **Joint Lubrication:**
Water contributes to the synovial fluid that lubricates joints, reducing friction and supporting smooth joint movement. Hydration is crucial for joint health and flexibility.

4. **Nutrient Transportation:**
Water acts as a medium for transporting nutrients throughout the body. It helps dissolve minerals, vitamins, and other essential substances, facilitating their absorption and distribution.

5. **Digestion and Absorption:**
Water aids in food digestion and absorption. It supports the breakdown of nutrients in the digestive system and helps transport them into the bloodstream for use by the body.

6. **Cognitive Function:**
Dehydration can have a negative impact on cognitive function, reducing concentration,

attentiveness, and short-term memory. Staying hydrated supports optimal brain function and mental clarity.

7. **Energy Production:**

Water is involved in the process of converting food into energy. Proper hydration ensures efficient energy production, reducing feelings of fatigue and supporting physical performance.

8. **Skin Health:**

Adequate hydration contributes to healthy skin by maintaining elasticity and preventing dryness. Dehydration can lead to skin issues, including premature aging and a lackluster complexion.

9. **Detoxification:**

Water plays a crucial role in the body's natural detoxification processes, helping flush out waste products and toxins through urine. Hydration supports kidney function and overall detoxification.

10. **Blood Pressure Regulation:**

Proper hydration helps maintain blood volume and supports blood pressure regulation. Dehydration can lead to an increase in blood viscosity, potentially affecting cardiovascular health.

11. **Exercise Performance:**

Hydration is critical for athletes and those who participate in strenuous activity. It helps prevent

dehydration, muscle cramps, and supports
endurance and performance during exercise.

12. **Mood and Stress Regulation:**
Dehydration can impact mood and increase
stress levels. Staying hydrated promotes emotional
well-being and helps the body better cope with
stress.

13. **Prevention of Heat-Related Illnesses:**
In hot climates or during strenuous activities,
staying hydrated is crucial for preventing
heat-related illnesses such as heatstroke or heat
exhaustion.

14. **Weight Management:**
Drinking water before meals can contribute to a
feeling of fullness, potentially reducing overall
calorie intake and supporting weight management
efforts.

15. **General Well-Being:**
Hydration is fundamental to overall well-being. It
contributes to various physiological processes,
helping the body function optimally and promoting
good health.

Ensuring regular and adequate water intake is
essential for maintaining health and supporting the
body's numerous functions. Individual hydration
requirements vary depending on age, exercise
intensity, climate, and overall health. Listening to

the body's thirst cues is a simple yet effective way
to maintain proper hydration.

ADJUSTING CARB INTAKE

Adjusting Carb Intake:

1. **Assess Individual Goals:**
   Consider your specific health and fitness goals.
Whether it's weight loss, muscle gain, or overall
well-being, your carb intake should align with your
objectives.

2. **Activity Level:**
   Modify your carb consumption, depending on
how active you are. Athletes and those with high
physical activity may require more carbohydrates
for energy, while sedentary individuals may need
fewer.

3. **Metabolic Health:**
   Individuals with certain metabolic conditions, such
as insulin resistance or diabetes, may benefit from
adjusting carb intake to manage blood sugar levels.
Consult a healthcare provider for personalized
advice.

4. **Body Composition:**
   Tailor carb intake to support your body
composition goals. For muscle building, consider
slightly higher carb intake, while those focusing on

fat loss may benefit from moderating carb
consumption.

5. **Dietary Preferences:**
Choose a carb intake that aligns with your dietary
preferences. Some individuals thrive on low-carb or
ketogenic diets, while others prefer a balanced
approach with moderate carb intake.

6. **Whole Foods vs. Processed Carbs:**
Prioritize whole, nutrient-dense carbs over
processed options. Whole grains, fruits, vegetables,
and legumes provide essential nutrients and fiber,
promoting overall health.

7. **Monitor Energy Levels:**
Pay attention to your energy levels and
performance. If you experience fatigue, low energy,
or performance issues, consider adjusting your
carb intake to ensure sufficient energy for daily
activities and workouts.

8. **Listen to Hunger and Fullness Cues:**
Tune in to your body's hunger and fullness
signals. Adjust carb intake based on how satisfied
you feel after meals, making sure you're not
overeating or undereating.

9. **Carb Cycling:**
Explore carb cycling, a strategy that involves
alternating between higher and lower carb days.
This approach can be beneficial for some

individuals, promoting fat loss while supporting muscle maintenance.

10. **Consider Macronutrient Ratios:**
Balance carb intake with proteins and fats. Adjust the ratios based on your nutritional needs and preferences. Some may thrive on a higher-carb, lower-fat diet, while others prefer a higher-fat, lower-carb approach.

11. **Adapt to Lifestyle Changes:**
Adjust your carb intake based on lifestyle changes. For example, if your activity level increases or decreases, consider modifying your carb consumption accordingly.

12. **Gradual Changes:**
Make gradual adjustments to carb intake. Sudden and drastic changes can be challenging to sustain. Give your body time to adapt and monitor how it responds.

13. **Consult a Professional:**
If uncertain about adjusting carb intake, seek guidance from a registered dietitian or nutritionist. They can provide personalized advice based on your individual needs, preferences, and health status.

Remember that there is no one-size-fits-all approach to carb intake, and what works for one person may not work for another. It's essential to find a balance that aligns with your individual goals, preferences, and overall well-being.

CHAPTER EIGHT

FITNESS AND CARB CYCLING

Points to note, during fitness and carb cycling:

1. **Aligning Carb Intake with Training Days:**
Adjust carb intake based on your workout schedule. On days with intense workouts, consider higher carb intake to fuel energy needs and support recovery.

2. **Timing Carbs Around Workouts:**
Consume a higher proportion of carbs around your workout window. This can enhance performance, replenish glycogen stores, and support muscle recovery.

3. **Higher Carbs on High-Intensity Days:**
Reserve higher carb days for high-intensity training sessions, such as strength training or HIIT. Carbs play a crucial role in providing quick energy during intense efforts.

4. **Moderate Carbs on Low-Intensity Days:**
On low-intensity or rest days, opt for moderate carb intake. Adjusting carb levels based on activity helps prevent excess calorie intake when energy expenditure is lower.

5. **Post-Workout Nutrition:**

Prioritize a combination of carbs and protein post-workout. This aids in glycogen replenishment and supports muscle repair and growth.

6. **Carb Cycling for Fat Loss:**

Some individuals use carb cycling as a strategy for fat loss. Alternating between higher and lower carb days can create a calorie deficit while preserving muscle mass.

7. **Individualized Approach:**

Fitness goals vary, and an individualized approach to carb cycling is crucial. Tailor your carb intake to your specific fitness objectives, whether it's muscle building, fat loss, or overall maintenance.

8. **Monitoring Performance:**

Pay attention to how your body responds to carb cycling. Monitor performance, energy levels, and recovery. Adjust the cycle based on what optimally supports your fitness endeavors.

9. **Adapt to Training Phases:**

Adapt carb cycling to different training phases. For instance, during a muscle-building phase, consider more frequent higher carb days, while during a fat loss phase, adjust accordingly.

10. **Balancing Macros:**

While carb cycling, ensure a balance of macronutrients. Include sufficient protein for muscle repair, and healthy fats for overall health and hormonal balance.

11. **Refeed Days:**

Incorporate periodic refeed days with higher carb intake. This can help prevent metabolic adaptation, replenish glycogen, and provide a psychological break from dieting.

12. **Stay Hydrated:**

Hydration is key for optimal performance. Maintain proper fluid intake, especially during workouts, to support endurance and recovery.

13. **Consult with a Professional:**

If unsure about implementing carb cycling in your fitness routine, consult with a nutritionist or dietitian. They can offer tailored advice depending on your needs and goals.

Remember, the effectiveness of carb cycling can vary among individuals. It's essential to experiment, monitor your body's response, and make adjustments based on your unique fitness goals and requirements.

TAILORING WORKOUT TO CARB CYCLE PHASES

Tailoring Workout to Carb Cycle Phases:

1. **High Carb Days:**
   - *Workout Focus:* Prioritize high-intensity workouts on these days, such as strength training or intense cardio. The increased carb intake provides readily available energy for optimal performance.

2. **Moderate Carb Days:**
   - *Workout Focus:* Engage in moderate-intensity workouts like moderate cardio or circuit training. The moderate carb intake supports sustained energy levels without the need for the same level of glycogen replenishment.

3. **Low Carb Days:**
   - *Workout Focus:* Consider focusing on lighter activities or restorative exercises on low carb days. This might include yoga, flexibility training, or low-intensity cardio. The body relies more on stored fat for energy during these sessions.

4. **Pre-Workout Nutrition:**
   - *High Carb Days:* Consume a balanced meal with a higher proportion of carbs 1-2 hours before the workout.
   - *Moderate Carb Days:* Include a mix of carbs and protein before the workout.

  - *Low Carb Days:* Opt for a lighter pre-workout snack with a focus on protein and healthy fats.

5. **Intra-Workout Nutrition:**
  - *High Carb Days:* Consider consuming a carbohydrate-rich drink during longer or more intense workouts.
  - *Moderate and Low Carb Days:* Hydration and electrolytes become crucial. Focus on maintaining adequate fluid balance during these sessions.

6. **Post-Workout Nutrition:**
  - *High Carb Days:* Prioritize a post-workout meal rich in both carbs and protein to replenish glycogen stores and support muscle recovery.
  - *Moderate Carb Days:* Continue with a balanced post-workout meal, adjusting the carb content based on the intensity of the session.
  - *Low Carb Days:* Emphasize protein intake to support muscle repair. Carbohydrates can be consumed later in the day.

7. **Hydration:**
  - *All Phases:* Stay well-hydrated throughout the workout. Adequate fluid intake is essential for performance and recovery.

8. **Adjusting Intensity:**
  - *High Carb Days:* Push yourself with higher intensity workouts, taking advantage of the increased energy availability.

   - *Moderate Carb Days:* Maintain a consistent
but slightly moderated workout intensity.
   - *Low Carb Days:* Listen to your body, and if
needed, reduce intensity to accommodate lower
energy levels.

9. **Rest and Recovery:**
   - *All Phases:* Prioritize rest days strategically,
aligning them with low or moderate carb days.
Adequate rest is crucial for overall recovery.

10. **Individual Response:**
   - *Experiment and Monitor:* Individuals
respond differently to carb cycling. Experiment with
different workout intensities during each phase and
monitor how your body responds. Adjust based on
your unique needs and performance.

11. **Professional Guidance:**
   - *Consult with a Trainer or Nutritionist:* Seek
advice from fitness professionals or nutritionists to
tailor the workout plan more precisely to your goals,
fitness level, and individual response to carb
cycling.

Remember, the key is to listen to your body,
monitor performance, and make adjustments as
needed. Individual preferences, fitness goals, and
responses to carb cycling may vary, so a
personalized approach is essential for optimizing
both workout and nutrition strategies.

RECOVERY NUTRITION

Recovery nutrition is crucial to replenish energy stores, repair muscle tissue, and support overall recovery after physical activity. Here's a comprehensive guide:

1. **Timing is Key:**

Consume a post-workout meal or snack within 30 to 60 minutes after exercise. This window is when the body is most receptive to nutrient absorption, aiding in glycogen replenishment and muscle repair.

2. **Protein Intake:**

Make protein a priority to aid with muscle synthesis and repair. Aim for a source of complete protein, such as lean meats, poultry, fish, eggs, dairy, or plant-based options like beans and legumes.

3. **Carbohydrates for Glycogen Replenishment:**

Consume carbs to restore the glycogen stores that were used up during activity. Choose complex carbs such as fruits, vegetables, and whole grains.

4. **Protein-to-Carb Ratio:**

Aim for a balanced protein-to-carbohydrate ratio in your recovery meal or snack. A common guideline is a 3:1 or 4:1 ratio of carbs to protein.

This helps maximize glycogen repletion and muscle protein synthesis.

5. **Hydration:**
Drink water or a beverage high in electrolytes to rehydrate. Proper hydration supports recovery, especially if the workout involves significant fluid loss through sweating.

6. **Electrolytes:**
Include electrolytes in your recovery plan, especially if the exercise was intense and led to electrolyte loss through sweat. Consider foods or drinks that contain potassium, sodium, magnesium, and calcium.

7. **Anti-Inflammatory Foods:**
Incorporate foods with anti-inflammatory properties, such as fruits, vegetables, fatty fish (rich in omega-3 fatty acids), and nuts. These can help mitigate exercise-induced inflammation.

8. **Micronutrients:**
Ensure your recovery nutrition includes a variety of micronutrients from colorful fruits and vegetables. This promotes overall health and aids in recovery processes.

9. **Snack Options:**
Opt for convenient and easily digestible snacks post-workout. Examples include a protein smoothie

with fruit, yogurt with granola, or a turkey sandwich on whole-grain bread.

10. **Whole Foods vs. Supplements:**
Whole meals offer a greater variety of nutrients, even though supplements can be more convenient. However, if immediate post-workout nutrition is challenging, a protein shake can be a convenient option.

11. **Individual Needs:**
Adjust the quantity and composition of your recovery nutrition based on the type, duration, and intensity of your exercise, as well as your individual goals and dietary preferences.

12. **Meal Composition:**
If your post-workout meal is a full meal, ensure it includes a balance of protein, carbohydrates, and healthy fats. For example, grilled chicken with quinoa and a side of vegetables.

13. **Consider Special Requirements:**
Individuals with specific dietary needs, such as vegetarians or those with food allergies, should consider alternatives that meet their nutritional requirements.

14. **Listen to Hunger Signals:**
Pay attention to hunger signals and adjust your recovery nutrition accordingly. If you're not hungry

immediately after exercise, consume a balanced meal within a reasonable timeframe.

15. **Consultation with a Professional:**
For personalized advice on recovery nutrition, especially for individuals with specific health conditions or performance goals, consult with a registered dietitian or nutritionist.

Recovery nutrition plays a pivotal role in optimizing performance, preventing fatigue, and supporting long-term fitness goals. Tailor your approach based on your unique needs and preferences, and consider seeking professional guidance for a personalized recovery plan.

CHAPTER NINE

FREQUENTLY ASKED QUESTIONS

1. What is carb cycling, and how does it work for women?

 - *Explanation:* Carb cycling involves alternating between higher and lower carbohydrate intake to optimize energy levels and potentially influence body composition. It works for women by providing a flexible approach to nutrition, syncing carb intake with activity levels and hormonal phases.

2. Can carb cycling help with weight loss for women?

 - *Explanation:* Yes, carb cycling can be a helpful strategy for weight loss in women. By creating a calorie deficit on lower carb days and optimizing nutrient timing, it may promote fat loss while preserving muscle mass.

3. How do I determine the right carb cycle for me?

 - *Explanation:* The right carb cycle depends on factors such as activity level, fitness goals, and individual response. Experiment with different ratios and cycle lengths, monitoring how your body responds, and adjust accordingly.

4. Is carb cycling suitable for all fitness levels?

   - *Explanation:* Carb cycling can be adapted to various fitness levels. It's important to tailor the approach to individual needs and preferences. Beginners may start with a simpler cycle, while advanced individuals might experiment with more intricate variations.

5. Are there risks associated with carb cycling for women?

   - *Explanation:* While carb cycling is generally safe, individuals with specific health conditions, such as diabetes or metabolic disorders, should consult with a healthcare professional before adopting this approach. It's crucial to monitor how your body responds and make adjustments as needed.

6. How can carb cycling benefit hormonal health in women?

   - *Explanation:* Carb cycling may benefit hormonal health by aligning carb intake with hormonal phases, supporting energy needs, and potentially mitigating the impact of prolonged low-carb diets on hormones like leptin and thyroid hormones.

7. Can I still build muscle with carb cycling?

   - *Explanation:* Yes, carb cycling can support muscle building. Higher carb days provide the energy needed for intense workouts, while lower carb days may promote fat loss, helping to reveal muscle definition.

8. What is the importance of macronutrient ratios in carb cycling?
   - *Explanation:* Macronutrient ratios, particularly balancing carbs, proteins, and fats, are crucial in carb cycling. They influence energy levels, muscle preservation, and overall effectiveness. Adjust ratios based on individual goals and preferences.

9. How does carb cycling align with different fitness goals, such as fat loss or muscle gain?
   - *Explanation:* Carb cycling can be adapted to different fitness goals. Higher carb days can support muscle gain, while lower carb days may create a calorie deficit, aiding fat loss. Individualization is key for optimal results.

10. Can I combine carb cycling with specific diets, like keto or vegetarianism?
   - *Explanation:* Yes, carb cycling can be combined with various diets, including keto or vegetarianism. It's essential to adjust carb levels based on the principles of the chosen diet and ensure nutritional needs are met.

Remember to consult with a healthcare professional or nutritionist when making significant changes to your diet, especially if you have underlying health conditions or specific dietary requirements.

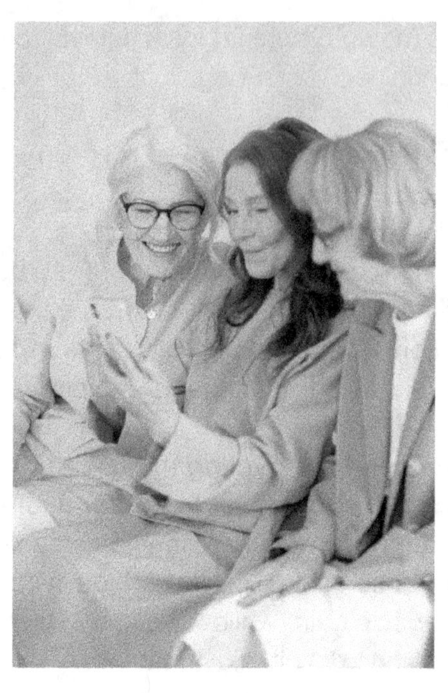

CONCLUSION

In conclusion, the Carb Cycling Cookbook for Women provides a comprehensive guide to harnessing the benefits of carb cycling for optimal health, fitness, and well-being. Through a carefully crafted approach to nutrition, this cookbook empowers women to align their carb intake with their unique physiology, activity levels, and fitness goals.

The cookbook begins by delving into the fundamentals of carb cycling, offering a nuanced understanding of how this approach can be tailored to women's specific needs. From setting macronutrient ratios to determining total daily caloric intake, the cookbook provides practical insights into the science and art of carb cycling.

One of the cookbook's strengths lies in its emphasis on the individualized nature of carb cycling. Recognizing that every woman is unique, the cookbook guides readers through the process of aligning carb cycling with their fitness goals, hormonal phases, and overall well-being. This personalized approach ensures that women can embrace carb cycling in a way that suits their lifestyles and aspirations.

The inclusion of detailed meal plans, recipes, and nutritional information further enhances the cookbook's practicality. Whether navigating high or low carb days, the cookbook offers a variety of delicious and nourishing options. From breakfast to dinner, snacks to desserts, each recipe is thoughtfully crafted to make carb cycling a flavorful and enjoyable journey.

As readers embark on their carb cycling adventure, the cookbook provides valuable insights into recovery nutrition, hydration, and adjusting carb intake. By addressing frequently asked questions and offering guidance on tailoring workouts to carb cycle phases, the cookbook becomes a holistic resource for women seeking to optimize their fitness and nutrition strategies.

In essence, the Carb Cycling Cookbook for Women stands as a supportive companion on the path to balanced and personalized nutrition. By combining science-backed information with practical and delectable recipes, this cookbook empowers women to embrace carb cycling as a sustainable and enjoyable way to achieve their health and fitness goals.

www.ingramcontent.com/pod-product-compliance
Lightning Source LLC
Chambersburg PA
CBHW070929260726
48661CB00003B/903